Cerebral Ischemia:

Clinical Implications and Therapeutics

Cerebral Ischemia:
Clinical Implications and Therapeutics

Edited by

**Robert H. Rosenwasser, Christer Carlsson
and Ronald F. Tuma**

Nova Science Publishers, Inc.

Art Director: Christopher Concannon
Graphics: Elenor Kallberg and Maria Ester Hawrys
Book Production: Michael Lyons, Roseann Pena,
                Casey Pfalzer, June Martino,
                Tammy Sauter, and Michelle Lalo
Circulation: Irene Kwartiroff, Annette Hellinger,
                and Benjamin Fung

Library of Congress Cataloging-in-Publication Data

Cerebral ischemia : clinical implications and therapeutics /
    edited by Robert H. Rosenwasser, Christer Carlsson,
    and Ronald F. Tuma.
        p. cm.
    Includes bibliographical references and index.
    ISBN 1-56072-137-5 : $62.00
    1. Cerebral ischemia.   I. Rosenwasser, Robert H.
  II. Carlsson, Christer. III. Tuma, Ronald F. (Ronald
  Franklin)
    [DNLM: 1. Cerebral Ischemia--physiology.
    2. Cerebral Ishemia--therapy.   WL 355 C41155 1993]
RC388.5.C3973   1993
616.8'1--dc20
DNLM/DLC   93-2122
for Library of Congress   CIP

© 1994 Nova Science Publishers, Inc.
  6080 Jericho Turnpike, Suite 207
  Commack, New York 11725
  Tele. 516-499-3103 Fax 516-499-3146
  E Mail Novasci1@aol.com

Printed in the United States of America

Table of Contents

Chapter 3.

Hemodynamic and Biochemical Implications of Vascular Cells in Cerebral Ischemia/Reperfusion: Future Directions and Treatment

Michelle C. Mazzoni and Karl-E. Arfors

Chapter 4.

Evaluation and Treatment of the Patient with an Acute Ischemic Infraction

Dara G. Jamieson

Chapter 5.

Guidelines for Anesthesia and Cerebral Protection in Neurovascular Surgery

Woodrow Wm. Wendling and Christer Carlsson

77

Chapter 6.

Critical Care Management of Neurovascular Problems in Patients Undergoing Non-Neurosurgical Procedures

Christer Carlsson and Woodrow Wm. Wendling

101

Chapter 7.

Critical Care Mangement of Neurovascular Problems: Practical and Theoretical Considerations　　111

Robert H. Rosenwasser

Chapter 8.

Morphologic Aspects of Cerebral Ischemia   165
Ehud Lavi and Dara G. Jamieson

INTRODUCTION

pproximately 500,000 new cases of stroke occur in the U.S. each year. Substantial progress has been made in the management of these patients. The recent explosion of information from research and clinical laboratories hold promise of significant advances in the future. Physicians in a wide variety of specialties encounter patients who have had or who are at risk for stroke. Therefore they must be aware of new developments in the understanding, prevention and treatment of cerebral infarcts. The primary goal of this book is to provide the practicing physician an updated survey of the latest knowledge concerning the pathophysiology and treatment of cerebral ischemia. Provided within this book is a review of the latest information available from both the research laboratory and the clinic. Every effort has been made to present information about the basic scientific principles related to cerebral ischemia in a format designed to be relevant and interesting to the practicing physician.

Current information about the normal physiologic control of cerebral blood flow along with a description of the pathophysiologic changes that are associated with cerebral ischemia are presented as a foundation and background for the sections dealing with the diagnosis and management of the patient suffering from ar at risk for cerebral ischemia. The management of the patient with or at risk for cerebral infarction is presented from the viewpoint of a variety of specialists, including a Neurologist, Neurosurgeon, Anesthesiologist and a Pathologist. Emphasis is placed on providing the background that enables the physician to understand the rationale behind pharmacologic approaches currently available as therapy for patients with cerebral ischemia. A similar background is presented for the understanding of the risks and benefits offered by surgical procedures performed on these patients.

The Office for Continuing Medical Education at Temple University School of Medicine provides opportunities for learning and relearning the knowledge, skills, and attitudes necessary for high quality medical care. One of the goals of this program is to help physicians keep informed of the latest theoretical and technical advances in medical science. This book attempts to help to fulfill this goal in the subject area of cerebral ischemia.

CME credit can be obtained through an examination based on the contents of this book.

DISCLOSURE POLICY:
It is the policy of Temple University School of Medicine, Office for Continuing Medical Education to insure balance, independence, objectivity and scientific rigor in all its sponsored educational programs. All faculty participating in sponsored programs by Temple University School of Medicine are expected to disclose to the program audiences any real or apparent conflict(s) or interest related to the content of their presentations(s).

ACCREDITATION STATEMENT:
Temple University School of Medicine is accredited by the Accreditation Council for Continuing Medical Education (ACCME) to sponsor Continuing Medical Education for Physicians.

CERTIFICATION STATEMENT:
Temple University School of Medicine designates this CME activity for 6 credit hours in Category I of the Physicians' Recognition Award of the A.M.A.

1

CONTROL OF CEREBRAL BLOOD FLOW

Ronald F. Tuma, Ph.D.
Professor
Department of Physiology and Neurosurgery
Temple University School of Medicine
Philadelphia, PA

Usha S. Vasthare, Ph.D.
Assistant Professor
Department of Physiology and Neurosurgery
Temple University School of Medicine
Philadelphia, PA

Numerous concepts about the function of the cerebral vessels, and indeed the brain itself, have been entertained over the centuries. However, the idea that the brain is an organ of vital importance is a very old one. The observation that there are "pulsations of the brain during life" is published in the Smith Papyrus, one of the earliest written medical texts (seventh century B.C.). When tracing the development of our understanding of the function of the cerebral circulation, one finds the process was far from straightforward. One complication was that the ancient Egyptians and early Greeks did not differentiate among tendons, blood vessels and nerves. The words neuron and neurology are derived from the Greek word whose original meaning was tendon. Despite this confusion some very early insights were presented. In the sixth century BC Pythagoras characterized the brain as the organ of reasoning. One of his pupils, Alcmeon of Croton recognized the movement of blood in the veins and the importance of blood for mental function. He theorized that sleep was caused by the "retreat" of blood from the brain into the great veins and that death occurred when this retreat was permanent. Unfortunately, these concepts were not perpetuated and refined by Hippocrates and Aristotle. They believed that the brain was a large gland which functioned to cool and purify the blood. The brain was thought to release excess fluids and other materials by nasal discharge.

Galen (129-199), although responsible for the introduction of numerous erroneous ideas, did provide some interesting additional insights into the operation and function of the brain. These concepts dominated physiological thought for the next millennium and a half. Galen presented the idea that the brain was nourished by both arterial and venous blood. He thought that the venous blood originated in the liver and intestines and provided a "natural spirit" to the brain. The arteries delivered blood containing a "vital spirit" that came from air brought in through the trachea and transported to the lungs, pulmonary veins and the right ventricle where it was mixed with the blood. The brain then formed an "animal spirit" which was distributed to all of the muscles via the hollow nerves. The delivery, or restriction of delivery of this animal spirit was responsible for controlling contraction of the muscles.

During the Renaissance, progress was made in clarifying the anatomic structure of the cerebral circulation. It is interesting that although he had even less insight into cardiovascular physiology than Galen, Leonardo da Vinci recognized that cervical compression could produce unconsciousness or irreversible damage if the compression lasted for more than "the hundredth part of an hour."(8)

Today we recognize the critical dependence of the brain on cardiovascular homeostasis and its inability to tolerate ischemia. This inability to tolerate ischemia is reflected in the way cerebral blood flow is regulated. Local factors predominate in the control of cerebral vascular resistance, whereas autonomic and hormonal control predominate in the regulation of vascular resistance in most other organs of the body. Under emergency circumstance, blood flow will be sacrificed in organs more tolerant of ischemia in order to preserve the brain.

The hemodynamic principles that govern flow to other organs of the body of course also apply to the regulation of the cerebral circulation. The magnitude of blood flow through the cerebral vessels is determined by the ratio of the pressure gradient across the cerebral vasculature to the cerebral vascular resistance as described by Poiseuilles Law. Where ΔP is the pressure gradient across the vessels, R is the vessel radius, L the vessel length and π the blood viscosity.

Although the principles governing the flow of blood, as outlined by Poiseuilles equation apply to all organs of the body there are some special ramifications when relating this equation to the cerebral circulation. The pressure gradient (ΔP) across the vasculature is of course the driving force for blood flow through any organ. The brain is somewhat special however, in that it will, through a number of reflexes, modulate systemic blood pressure to levels that will help to ensure an adequate pressure gradient for it's survival. When cerebral blood flow is compromised by an elevation in cerebral spinal fluid pressure, reflexes are initiated that can increase systemic blood pressure to extraordinarily high levels.

Although vessel length (L) is something that is not a "regulated parameter", the morphometry of the cerebral vasculature imparts special significance to this parameter when applying Poiseuilles' equation to the brain. Cerebral arterial vessels are very long compared to similar arterial segments in other organs of the body. This results in the larger cerebral arterial vessels contributing more to vascular resistance in the brain than the same branching order in other organs. Large extracranial vessels contribute 60-70% of the total precapillary vascular resistance. In later sections it will be seen that this role of the larger arterial vessels will influence the way that sympathetic stimulation effects cerebral vascular resistance. The fact that large cerebral arterial vessels contribute significantly to resistance allows these vessels to counteract local "steal" phenomenon that would occur with regional increases in metabolic rate (6).

Blood viscosity becomes a factor of concern when considering the type of fluid replacement that should be used under various clinical circumstances. It is speculated that under certain conditions, the delivery of oxygen to the brain and other organs, may be optimized by lowering the hematocrit to values below normal (28%) while maintaining normal or slightly expanded blood volume (18).

The mechanisms responsible for the control of vessel radius also have specific adaptations in the brain, reflecting the critical need for uninterrupted blood supply. In all organs of the body the algebraic sum of the factors that are involved in the control of smooth muscle tone determine the final resting diameter of the resistance vessels. These factors can be divided into systemic and local control mechanisms. Systemic mechanisms are directed at the regulation of systemic blood pressure, whereas the local control mechanisms are directed at the regulation of blood flow at a level commensurate with tissue needs. Systemic control mechanisms can be divided into hormonal and neural control mechanisms. Local control mechanisms can be subdivided into myogenic, metabolic and endothelial control.

NEURAL CONTROL

There are four components of the nervous system that have the potential to influence vascular diameter: sympathetic nerves, parasympathetic nerves, the central noradrenergic pathway, and sensory nerves. The possibilities for regulation of cerebrovascular resistance are extensive. Over fifteen vasoactive neurotransmitters have been demonstrated in axons innervating blood vessels in the Circle of Willis, including peptides and biogenic amines (14).

The response of the cerebral vessels to sympathetic stimulation differs significantly from the response of vessels in other organs of the body. Adrenergic receptors on the smooth muscle of the cerebral resistance vessels are less dense and less sensitive to stimulation compared to the adrenergic receptors on the resistance vessels in other organs of the body. The ED_{50} for norepinephrine is one hundred times greater for the basilar artery than for the saphenous artery. Adrenergic receptor stimulation in cerebral vessels also appear to lead to greater calcium influx from the extracellular fluid, which leads to interesting speculation about selective effects of calcium channel blockers on cerebral vasculature (11,17). The results of sympathetic stimulation on cerebral vascular resistance are influenced by the fact that the larger cerebral vessels are much more responsive to stimulation than the small cerebral arterial vessels. The relative contribution of the large vs. small cerebral arterial vessels differs when systemic blood pressure changes. Under conditions of hypertension larger cerebral vessels contribute more to vascular resistance in the brain whereas under hypotensive conditions the smaller cerebral vessels contribute more to resistance. Since the sympathetic nerves have a greater influence over the larger vessels, sympathetic stimulation increases resistance when blood pressure increases, but has little effect on cerebral vascular resistance under when blood pressure is low. This is very beneficial with regard to homeostasis of the brain because sympathetic stimulation will help protect the capillaries from exposure to high pressures when blood pressure increases, protecting the blood brain barrier. At the same time, because of the lack of effect on smaller cerebral arterioles, sympathetic stimulation contributes very little to cerebrovascular resistance when there is a significant reduction in blood pressure. The fact that sympathetic stimulation does not increase cerebrovascular resistance when there is a reduction in mean blood pressure allows for a preferential redistribution of the cardiac output to the brain under hypotensive conditions. Sympathetic nerves also seem to have a trophic effect on cerebral vessels, promoting vascular hypertrophy (5). As described below this may have significant effects on long term autoregulatory adaptations in the brain.

The role of parasympathetic nerves in the regulation of cerebral blood flow is still unclear. Probable sites of origin of parasympathetic nerves innervating the cerebral blood vessels are the sphenopalatine ganglion, the otic ganglia and internal carotid miniganglia (20). Parasympathetic nerve terminals in the CNS costore Ach and vasoactive intestinal peptide (VIP). Parasympathetic nerves also release peptide histidine isoleucine (PHI) which is synthesized from the same precursor as VIP, prepoVIP, and in some cases neuropeptide Y (1,2,20). VIP acts directly on smooth muscle cell VIP receptors, inducing an endothelial cell independent relaxation that has a greater effect on small arterial vessels than large arterial vessels (2). It has been speculated that the parasympathetic nervous system may participate in the development of collateral flow. This speculation is based on the observation that parasympathetic denervation increases infarct size in focal but not global ischemic models, indicating that flow may be better preserved in the penumbra when the parasympathetic nerves are intact (14).

Recent studies have provided evidence for important contributions of sensory nerve fibers in the regulation of cerebral blood flow (12-14). Included among the ganglia receiving projections from these sensory nerves are the trigeminal ganglia, internal carotid miniganglia and cervical dorsal root ganglia. Peripheral ramifications of primary sensory (type C unmyleninated) neurons are thought to release a number of vasoactive neuropeptides. Two of the major vasoactive neuropeptides released by sensory neurons are substance P (SP) and calcitonin gene related peptide (CGRP). These neurons also release a second tachykinin neurokinin A. The relaxation caused by release of SP and NKA is dependent upon the presence of functioning endothelial cells, whereas vasorelaxation induced by CGRP release is both more potent and endothelial independent. A number of functions have been proposed for these sensory nerves. In animals studies, trigeminal ganglion lesion has been demonstrated to prolong the vasoconstrictor responses to elevated pH, $PGF_{2\alpha}$, and superfused norepinephrine are prolonged. It has therefore been postulated that CGRP is involved in the restoration of normal vascular diameter under conditions of intense vasoconstriction such as subarachnoid hemorrhage (1, 2). In a cat model it has been demonstrated that trigeminal ganglionectomy prolongs vasoconstriction caused by perivascular blood injection. The same investigator reports that there is depletion of CGRP but not of other perivascular neuropeptides in patients who have died following subarachnoid hemorrhage. CGRP depletion has also been reported in a rat model of subarachnoid hemorrhage (1). The enhanced concentration of CGRP in the external jugular vein during migraine headache has also lead to speculation that these sensory nerves may also be linked to this problem.

These neurons may also play an important role in reactive hyperemia following transient cerebral ischemia. Trigeminal ganglionectomy has been reported to reduce reactive hyperemia following 10 min of global ischemia in cats by almost 50% (13-15). These investigators speculate that blocking this mechanism may be a useful strategy in reducing severe cortical hyperemia.

Very little is understood about the functional significance of the central noradrenergic pathway, originating in the locus cerileus. There is no current evidence for involvement in the regulation of cerebral blood flow, but it is speculated that these neurons may influence capillary permeability.

The final potential role of nerves in the regulation of cerebral blood flow involves the coupling of increased metabolic demand of the neurons with increased blood flow. Pial arterioles are innervated by nerve fibers from bipolar neurons within the cerebral cortex. These fibers contain VIP and PHI.

It is possible that the release of these peptides could elicit vasodilation when tissue metabolism increases (20).

LOCAL CONTROL MECHANISMS

METABOLIC CONTROL

In 1890 Roy and Sherrington postulated that the chemical products of metabolism can cause variations in the calibre of cerebral blood vessels (15). This mechanism, which provides the precise coupling between the metabolic requirements of the brain parenchyma and the magnitude of blood flow, predominates under normal circumstances. Precise coupling is essential since reductions in flow by as little as 40% can produce significant alterations in cerebral function. The cerebral resistance vessels are responsive to a number of metabolites. Increasing interstitial fluid concentration of hydrogen ions, carbon dioxide, potassium, adenosine or decreasing the partial pressure of oxygen all result in a relaxation of vascular smooth muscle and dilation of the cerebral resistance vessels. There is continuing debate as to the relative importance of each of these metabolites in the normal regulation of cerebral blood flow.

It has been postulated by a number of investigators (6) that adenosine is the primary metabolite involved in metabolic control. Adenosine is produced as a byproduct of ATP metabolism when oxygen delivery to the cells is insufficient to maintain energy stores. ATP is metabolized to ADP, AMP and then through the action of a 5'C'-nucleotidase to adenosine which diffuses into the interstitial fluid. Adenosine is thought to stimulate A_2 receptors on smooth muscle cells (7). This stimulation results in a decrease in cytosolic calcium in vascular smooth muscle and therefore vasodilation.

Although it is not strictly a byproduct of metabolism, the concentration of potassium in the interstitial fluid of the brain increases with increase in neuronal activity. Potassium is lost from the cytosol of neurons during depolarization. Increases in potassium concentration between 1-10 mM cause hyperpolarization of vascular smooth muscle through an inducible electrogenic pump on the cell membrane and relaxation of vascular smooth muscle. Potassium initially received considerable attention because it was felt that its interstitial accumulation might precede that of adenosine and therefore explain the initial hyperemic response to elevations in metabolic rate. There are however questions (10) as to whether the vasodilator effect of potassium on smooth muscle is rapid enough to explain this initial hyperemic response. The finding that amphetamines increase cerebral blood flow without any detectable effect on potassium concentration also casts doubt on the predomonance of potassium in the regulation of cerebral blood flow.

Increases in the metabolic rate of the brain, if not matched by an increase in blood flow, also results in an increase in both CO_2 and hydrogen ion concentration. The prominent vasodilation of the cerebral vessels in response to hypercapnia has been well recognized for many years. It has been clearly established that CO_2 does not directly influence vascular smooth muscle, but rather operates indirectly through changes in hydrogen ion concentration (6). Hydrogen ions are unable to cross the blood brain barrier, but CO_2 which is very lipid soluble, crosses the blood brain barrier freely. The resultant decrease in pH in the extracellular fluid then causes dilation of the pial arterial vessels. Small pial arterial vessels dilate more than larger vessels, probably because the larger vessels are also influenced by reflex sympathetic stimulation that occurs during hypercapnia (19). With chronic hypercapnia or hypocapnia, the bicarbonate concentration of the CSF changes and therefore blunts the effect of altered blood CO_2 on cerebral vessels.

Hypoxia also causes cerebral vasodilation. The influence of alterations in blood oxygen tension is often misunderstood because hypoxia is often accompanied by hyperventilation. The reduction in CO_2 tends to cause constriction of the cerebral vessels and mask the dilation resulting from hypoxia. When not accompanied by changes in CO_2 cerebral blood flow is linearly related to alterations in arterial blood oxygen content. It is unlikely that changes in tissue PO_2 directly effects vascular smooth muscle, but probably has its effect through changes in adenosine production.

The major question that has been raised about the predominant role of adenosine, or other metabolites, in providing the coupling between cerebral metabolism and cerebral blood flow relates to the rapidity with which cerebral vascular diameter changes when metabolism is altered in the brain. Fox and Raichle (3) studied the effect of somatosensory stimulation on cerebral blood flow, cerebral oxygen consumption and oxygen extraction in humans using PET. These investigators found that cerebral blood flow increases more than cerebral metabolism within one to two seconds after stimulation. There are also a number of pathophysiological situations such as hyperthermia and status epilepticus during which cerebral blood flow increases more than the metabolic requirements. Lou et al. (10) postulate that a neuronal reflex is responsible for the initial vasodilation that accompanies an increase in metabolism. It is of course possible that there are separate mechanisms responsible for the initial increase in blood flow in response to an increase in metabolism and for the maintenance of flow with a sustained elevation in metabolic rate. Adenosine, if not able to totally explain the initial increase in flow, is a likely candidate as the factor responsible for the sustained effect.

ENDOTHELIAL CONTROL

At one time endothelial cells were viewed to be principally a passive barrier that restricted the transport of macromolecules between the plasma and the interstitial fluid. Today we know that these small cells are centrally involved in a number of physiologic and pathophysiologic responses. As discussed in Chapter 3, endothelial cells can express adhesion molecules on their surface to signal platelets and leukocytes to adhere under certain circumstances. Another important role is the release of vasoactive mediators that may play a significant role in the regulation of vascular resistance. The role of endothelial cells in the regulation of blood flow is a subject that has received considerable attention during the last decade. This has shed new light upon our understanding of the regulation of blood flow under both physiologic and pathophysiologic conditions.

The observation that blood vessels dilated when exposed to ACh in-vivo but isolated muscle rings constricted when exposed to ACh in-vitro was made in numerous laboratories. Although contradictory, these results received little attention. The situation changed when Furchgott and Zawadzki demonstrated that the constrictor response to ACh in-vitro occurred when the endothelial cells were removed from the blood vessels, as was usually the case with most in-vitro preparations (4). They showed that vasodilation was also occurred in-vitro when the endothelial lining of the vessels was left intact. They therefore were the first to propose that the endothelial cells produced a vasoactive substance that could affect the contractile tone of vascular smooth muscle. These findings stimulated numerous intensive investigations of endothelial function, and led to the discovery of a number of endothelial derived vasoactive substances. Today we know that endothelial cells produce at least six different vasoactive substances that are thought to be involved in the regulation of vascular diameter under both physiological and pathophysiologic conditions.

There are at least three different substances produced by endothelial cells that cause relaxation of blood vessels: endothelium derived relaxing factor (EDRF), prostacycline and endothelium derived hyperpolarizing factor (EDHF).

The major dilator produced by the endothelial cells is EDRF. EDRF is thought to be nitric oxide, a free radical. Exposure of smooth muscle cells to EDRF increases cyclic GMP levels leading to relaxation. The fact that EDRF is a free radical is important since this property makes it very short acting. Since it is a free radical it is rapidly destroyed by superoxide anions and protected by a number of antioxidant substances (such as Vitamin E). EDRF also reacts readily with hemoglobin Therefore the presence of hemoglobin in the interstitial fluid, such as may occur after hemorrhage, may inactivate EDRF.

EDHF differs from EDRF in the way that it influences smooth muscle cells. Whereas EDRF causes relaxation by increasing cGMP levels, EDHF causes relaxation by hyperpolarizing the cell membrane, as its name implies.

The third dilator produced is the prostacycline (PGI_2). Prostacycline is a derivative of arachidonic acid through the cycloxygenase pathway. Although it does function as a vasodilator, the most important effect of PGI_2 is probably its inhibitory effect on platelet aggregation. The paracrine function of the endothelial cells is very important in helping to restrict the constricting action of platelets and helping to prevent unwanted aggregation. Since endothelial cells may attenuate the reaction of the blood vessel to substances released by the platelets, they probably have an important role in protecting the vessel from atherosclerosis. Alterations in endothelial function may therefore have both immediate and very long term effects.

The stimuli that induce the release of endothelial derived relaxing substances are shear stress, locally produced autocoids such as histamine bradykinin, substance P and factors released from platelets. The response of the endothelial cells to shear stress may have particular significance for the regulation of cerebral circulation. Flow induced vasodilation of large cerebral vessels may help counteract cerebral steal syndrome.

In addition to the vasodilating substances there are also at least three different vasoconstrictors produced by endothelial cells. One of the endothelial derived contracting factors requires functioning cyclooxygenase. A second contracting factor released by endothelial cells remains to be identified. This factor appears to be released by anoxic endothelial cell. The response is very rapid in onset and poorly sustained. A third constricting factor released by endothelial cells is the peptide endothelin. The contraction induced by endothelin is very slow in onset and long in duration. Cerebral vessels are especially sensitive to endothelin. The fact that endothelin can cause contractions of such long duration has lead to speculation that this factor may be involved in the pathogenesis of cerebral vasospasm. The contraction in response to endothelin is mediated by activation of nimodipine sensitive calcium channels. This presents interesting therapeutic implications.

It appears therefore that endothelial cells are able to release a number of substances that can cause either relaxation or constriction of smooth muscle cells. Under normal conditions the balance of factors released appears to favor vasodilation, whereas under a number of pathological conditions this balance is shifted toward the release of constricting factors.

MYOGENIC CONTROL

Cerebral blood vessels have been demonstrated to be myogenically active. The myogenic response is independent of endothelial cells. The controlled parameter in the myogenic response is vascular wall tension. By normalizing wall tension when there is an increase in transluminal pressure the vessels will decrease their radius, increase resistance to blood flow and help protect the capillaries against elevations in pressure.

AUTOREGULATION

The effectiveness of local control mechanisms is reflected in the autoregulatory ability of the cerebral vasculature. The cerebral vessels are capable of keeping blood flow constant when perfusion pressures range between 60 and 140 mmHg. The ability to autoregulate at the high pressure range is enhanced by sympathetic stimulation. Since sympathetic stimulation only causes constriction of the large arterial vessels when they are exposed to high pressure, sympathetic stimulation has little influence when blood pressure drops. The autoregulatory range is influenced by chronic alterations in pressure. Hypertensive individuals respond to the increase in pressure by hypertrophy of the wall of the cerebral arterial vessel. This results in an enhanced ability to regulate blood pressure in the high pressure range but a decrease in the ability maintain flow constant in the face of reductions in blood pressure.

SUMMARY

Recent investigations have brought to light a substantial amount of information about potential mechanisms for the regulation of cerebral blood flow. Although our knowledge has increased considerably about each of these control mechanisms, the way in which these mechanisms interact in the intact system is still not well understood. The relative importance of these various control mechanisms under various circumstances remains to be determined.

REFERENCES

1.   Edvinsson, L., Delgado-Zygmunt, T., Ekman, R., Jansen, I., Svendgaard, N.A. and Uddman, R.: Involvement of perivascular sensory fibers in the pathophysiology of cerebral vasospasm following subarachnoid hemorrhage. *J Cereb. Blood Flow Metab.* 10:602-607, 1990.

2.   Edvinsson, L.: Innervation and effects of dilatory neuropeptides on cerebral blood vessels. *Blood Vessels* 28:35-45, 1991

3.   Fox, P.T., Raichle, M.E.: Focal physiological uncoupling of cerebral blood flow and oxidative metabolism during somatosensory stimulation in human subjects. *Proc Natl Acad Sci USA* 83:1140-1144, 1986.

4.   Furchgott, R.F., and Zawadzki, J.V. The obligatory role of endothelial cells in the relaxation of arterial smooth muscle by acetylcholine. *Nature* 299: 373-376, 1980.

5.   Hart, M.D., Heistad, D.D., and Brody, M.J.: Effect of chronic hypertension and sympathetic denervation on wall/lumen ratio of cerebral arteries. *Hypertension* 2:410-423, 1980.

6.   Heistad, D.D. and Kontos, H.A.: Cerebral Circulation in <u>Handbook of Physiology; Section 2: The Cardiovascular System</u> (J.T. Shepherd and F.M Abbout, eds.) American Physiological Society. pp 137-182, 1983

7.   Ibayashi, S., Ngai, A.C., Meno, J.R. and Winn, H.R.: Effects of topical adenosine analogs and forskolin on rat pial arterioles in-vivo. *J. Cereb. Blood Flow Metab.* 11:72-76, 1991.

8.   Kety, S.S.: The Cerebral Circulation in <u>Circulation of the Blood; Men and Ideas</u> (A.P. Fishman and D.W. Richards(eds)). Oxford University Press. 1964 pp. 703-742.

9.   Kozniewska, E., Oseka, M., and Stys, T.: Effects of endothelium-derived nitric oxide on cerebral circulation during normoxia and hypoxia in the rat. *J. Cereb. Blood Flow Metab.* 12:311-317, 1992.

10.   Lou, H.C., Edvinsson, L. and E.T. MacKenzie, : The concept of coupling blood flow to brain function: Revision Required? *Ann Neurol* 22:289-297, 1987

11.   McCalden, T.A. and Bevan, J.A.: Sources of activator calcium in rabbit basilar artery. *Am. J. Physiol.* 241:H129-H133, 1981.

12.   Macfarlane, R., Moskowitz, M.A., Tasdemiroglu, E., Wei, E.P. and Kontos, H.A.: Postischemic cerebral blood flow and neuroeffector mechanisms. *Blood Vessels* 28:46-51, 1991.

13.   Macfarlane, R., Tasdemiroglu, E., Moskowitz, A., Uemura, Y., Wei, E.P. and Kontos, H.: Chronic trigeminal ganglionectomy or topical capsaicin application to pial vessels attenuates postocclusive cortical hyperemia but does not influence postischemic hypoperfusion. *J Cereb. Blood Flow Metab.* 11:261-271, 1991.

14.   Moskowitz, M.A., Macfarlane, R., Tasdemiroglu, E., Wei, E.P. and Kontos, H.A.: Neurogenic control of the cerebral circulation during global ischemia. *Stroke* 21:III168-171, 1990.

15   Roy, C.W., Sherrington, C.S.: On the regulation of the blood supply of the brain. J Physiol (London) 11:85-108, 1890.

16.   Rosenblum, W.I., Nishimura, H. and Nelson, G.H.: Endothelium-dependent L-Arg and L- NMA-sensitive mechanisms regulate tone of brain microvessels. *Am J Physiol* 259:H1396- H1401, 1990.

17.   Towart, R.: The selective inhibition of serotonin-induced contractions of rabbit vascular smooth muscle by calcium antagonistic dihydropyridines. An investigation of the mechanism of action of nimodipine. *Circ. Res.* 48: 650-657, 1981.

18.   Tuma, R.F., J.V. White, and Messmer, K (eds.): <u>The Role of Hemodilution in Optimal Patient Care</u> .W. Zuckschwerdt Verlag 1989.

19.   Wei, E.P., Kontos, H.A., and Patterson, J.L.: Dependence of pial arteriolar response to hypercapnia on vessel size. *Am J. Physiol* 238(Heart Circ Physiol. 7): H697-H703, 1980.

20.   Zhang, E-T., Mikkelsen, J.D., Fahrenkrug, J., Moller, M., Kronborg, D. and Lauritzen, M.: Prepo-vasoactive intestinal polypeptide-derived peptide sequences in cerebral blood vessels of rats: On the functional anatomy of metabolic autoregulation. *J. Cereb. Blood Flow Metab.* 11:932-938, 1991.

2

PATHOPHYSIOLOGY OF ISCHEMIA AND REPERFUSION: BASIC CONCEPTS

Usha S. Vasthare, Ph.D.
Assistant Professor
Department of Physiology and Neurosurgery
Temple University School of Medicine
Philadelphia, PA

Robert H. Rosenwasser, M.D., F.A.C.S.
Associate Professor of Neurological Surgery
and Physiology
Director, Neurological Intensive Care Unit
Temple University Hospital
Philadelphia, PA

INTRODUCTION

At one time it was felt that the brain has limited tolerance to ischemic damage simply because neurons have minimal levels of stored metabolic substrates and therefore very little potential for anaerobic metabolism. The factors responsible for limited tolerance of the brain appear to be however, much more complicated. Studies from the 1960's (1) showing extensive recovery of retinal neurons in vitro following anoxia lead us to believe that vascular factors may be involved in the damage. Another major concept that stemmed from studies in 1960's is that many of the pathological changes occur not only during the ischemic episode but also during reperfusion. This accentuation of ischemic damage during reperfusion period is now termed as "Reperfusion Injury." The clinical importance of this Reperfusion Injury is overwhelming since it allows for potential therapeutic interventions.

The damage that occurs in the brain following ischemia can be divided into two general categories. The pathogenesis of such kind of damage is different. If the insult is mild enough, there is Selective Neuronal Necrosis without affecting glial and vascular cells(55,67). The other type of damage will lead to infarction which includes all cell types (Pan Necrosis)(28,52).

The duration of ischemia is one of the major determining factors for this pathogenesis(55,67). The other major determining factor that determines whether the damage will affect only the neurons or further lead to infarction, is the nutritional state of the brain tissue (53,60,61).

There are three zones of hemodynamic and metabolic function which must be considered in the discussion of cerebral ischemic events. First is the central zone of ischemic tissue, which is ultimately destined for infarction, and unless intervention is immediate has no chance of recovery. Second is the border zone, which is questionably idling tissue whose fate may be either death and infarction or recovery. The collateral zone is the tissue which retains its viability and is frequently hyperemic. The central zone has zero to minimal flow and, in general, is less than 10 cc/100 grams/minute. There is associated massive influx of sodium and water with low tissue oxygen content and low tissue pH. The border zone, or ischemic penumbra, has flows of 10-15 cc/100 grams/minute and metabolically may remain viable (3,4,17), however, neurophysiologically, it is electrically silent. In this region ATP is maintained for membrane viability, but is insufficient to maintain levels of creatine phosphate and low levels of lactate.

The term ischemic penumbra was first described by Astrup et al in 1981(3), and was defined as the tissue zone lying peripheral to the region of dense ischemia. In the ischemic penumbra, the cerebral blood flow decrement has exceeded the threshold for failure of electrical function; however, as previously stated, the ion pump and membrane permeability and stability are maintained (37). Tissue water content is essentially unchanged from control values. It is in the ischemic penumbra, or in the area of the ischemic penumbra, that therapeutic intervention may be undertaken to restore flow and homeostasis to prevent the so-called secondary injury. Early measures to enhance collateral circulation and perfusion might avert acute injury triggered by further hemodynamic failure. In the ischemic penumbra, cerebral oxygen extraction, particularly in models of human stroke, is elevated with an associated decrease in cerebral blood flow, sometimes termed "misery perfusion." (6-11) This is ultimately followed by a decrease in the cerebral oxygen extraction fraction, when infarction is imminent. Positron emission tomographic studies have indicated that there are local elevations in the oxygen extraction fraction in the face of diminished perfusion, observed in the first hours after the primary ictus. Misery perfusion denotes the attempt of the tissue threatened by ischemia to continue oxidative metabolism despite limitations of perfusion.

The following sections deals with the putative role of various factors that are postulated to be involved in the genesis of cerebral ischemic damage. Although these factors are discussed separately for the sake of simplicity and clarity, it should be recognized that these factors are mutually inclusive. These factors are inter dependent and inter related to such an extent that no drug with single mode of action can be used to attenuate the damage.

ACIDOSIS

Ischemia, leads to an increased tissue lactate content and thereby reduction in pH(62). During complete ischemia, the magnitude of acidosis correlates closely to preischemic tissue stores of glucose and glycogen. Thus hypoglycemia is associated with less lactic acid production and consequently less reduction in pH whereas hyperglycemia is associated with increased lactic acid production and greater reduction in pH. Myers and co-workers first described findings that elevated blood glucose markedly altered the pathological response of the cerebral tissue to ischemic events (47,48). This was demonstrated in food deprived monkeys submitted to 14 minutes of cardiac arrest, which showed minimal or no signs of neuropathological change, whereas brains of monkeys which had been fed glucose demonstrated widespread neuronal and glial pathological changes. Pulsinelli and co-workers demonstrated that when glucose was given before or during the ischemic period, the cellular damage noted on pathological examination had increased (54,55). Glucose given after the ischemic event failed to influence the neuropathological outcome. These authors also reported, in an animal model, that a two- to threefold increase in pre-ischemic and ischemic glucose concentration was sufficient to increase the number of damaged neurons in the striatum, cerebellum, hippocampus and selectively to certain neurons in the cerebral cortex.

During incomplete ischemia, the magnitude of reduction in pH is far greater than in complete ischemia because of continued delivery of glucose by the residual blood flow. Thus the seemingly paradoxical finding that the magnitude of damage that occurs after complete cessation of blood flow is often less severe than if ischemia is incomplete with a trickle of flow still remaining can be explained by the fact that there is increased production of lactic acid and increased levels of hydrogen ion concentration and thereby greater reduction in pH during incomplete ischemia. It was demonstrated that if the animals were fasted for a day before inducing incomplete ischemia, there was no longer any difference in the magnitude of damage that occurred in these animals when compared to animals with complete interruption of flow (60).

Although the mechanism of glucose mediated neuronal and glial damage has been studied by many investigators, the molecular mechanism of membrane dysfunction as a result of increases in hydrogen ion concentration during ischemia is not very clear. It is speculated that failure of normalization of pHe inhibits Na/H antiporter and consequently the normalization of pHi. This eventually leads to osmolytic damage of neurons and compression of the microvasculature. It is believed that glial cells may play a role in buffering hydrogen ions; however, during severe ischemia there is also failure of the glia which becomes a vicious cycle as the pH is continuously depressed. However, the role of non-neuronal tissue in pH regulation is highly controversial.

The effect of acidosis is possibly compounded by the fact that it may lead to dislocation of protein bound iron from transferrin and ferritin leading to potentiation of free radical formation via hydroxyl radical generation. (5,57,63)

ROLE OF CALCIUM

Calcium plays an important role as both a second messenger and metabolic regulator. Calcium can also mediate ischemic cell death. When cyotosolic calcium levels increase, calcium complexes with calmodulin. The calcium-calmodulin complex can cause activation of a number of enzymes that can have detrimental effects on the cell. Activation of phospholipase A_2 occurs causing the release of free fatty acids, including arachidonic acid, from the cell membrane. Activation of phosphatidylinositol phosphodiestrase can also occur, which then breaks the envelop surrounding the neurotransmitters and potentiates their release (19,32,36,46). Activation of calcium dependent proteases and lipases can result in disruption of not only the membrane but also the cytoskeleton.

These processes continue until calcium is sequestered by the mitochondria and endoplasmic reticulum. Calcium ATPase is responsible for calcium removal from the cytoplasm and is activated by an increased cytosolic content of calcium. The methods of calcium removal are energy dependent. With depleted energy stores that occur during ischemia, the transport of calcium across leaking mitochondrial membranes occurs, with an uncoupling of oxidative phosphorylation. This becomes a vicious cycle with essential disruption of cell membranes due to mitochondrial failure. There are numerous studies demonstrating that calcium antagonists attenuate ischemic and reperfusion injury.(64)

Even though it is clearly demonstrated that continued increases in intracellular calcium will eventually lead to cell death, it is not well established whether increased intracellular calcium is the primary causative factor for ischemic damage or whether it just promotes the damage initiated by other factors.

It was previously assumed that calcium entered cells via the Voltage Sensitive Calcium Channels (VSCC) only, which were believed to be present in apical dendrites. However, it is now demonstrated that Calcium can also enter the cell via the Agonist Operated Calcium Channels (AOCC) especially those stimulated by the excitatory neurotransmitters. It is also established based on the studies on peripheral neurons that there are at least three different types of VSCC's viz; L (Long lasting), T (Transient) and N (Neither L nor T) type channels(50). It is believed that the conventional calcium antagonists like the Dihydropyridine derivatives block the L type channels. Recently, a hypothesis was put forward by Seisjo and Bengston (64) which explains that the presynaptic calcium influx is through VSCC (probably the N type) which is not blocked by conventional calcium channel blockers. This presynaptic calcium influx causes neurotransmitter release.

These excitatory neurotransmitter receptors (Kainate, Quisqualate and NMDA) on the post synaptic membrane when activated allow monovalent sodium and potassium ions and divalent calcium ions respectively.

The use of calcium channel blockers have elicited only moderate beneficial effects mostly in focal ischemic models. In severe ischemic models, there was a lack of marked protective effect by these calcium channel blockers (whether VSCC or AOCC). It may be that during severe ischemia, calcium can enter the cell by many different routes and that either VSCC blocker or AOCC blocker alone may not be able to ameliorate the calcium influx completely (64).

Of late, proponents of calcium hypothesis, have speculated that calcium could be responsible for selective vulnerability of neurons and for delayed neuronal death.

INVOLVEMENT OF LEUKOCYTES

Recently, leukocytes have been implicated to play an important role in cerebral ischemia and reperfusion injury. Experimental evidence suggest that leukocytes do indeed exacerbate injury that is caused during ischemia and reperfusion of the brain (14,21,31,69). There are many number of ways in which leukocytes could at least in theory, contribute to accentuating the damage that occurs during ischemia and reperfusion. First, is through simple mechanical occlusion or plugging of the capillaries. Under normal flow conditions, it takes about 700 times as much pressure to force a leukocyte through a capillary, albeit the fact that there are approximately 700 RBC's for each WBC. This is because the time taken for a leukocyte to deform itself is about 1000 times longer than for a RBC because of the presence of the nucleus. Under normal conditions this lack of deformability is not much of a problem because the pressure gradients that normally exist are adequate to force the leukocyte through the microvessels. However, under conditions of reduced perfusion pressure the capillaries may act like a sieve and trap the leukocytes. This degree of plugging that would occur could be enhanced if the capillary endothelium becomes swollen during and after an ischemic challenge.

In addition to the passive mechanical effects, a number of chemical mediators are released during ischemia that can lead to an increased number of circulating leukocytes and their activation. Activation can lead to enhanced adhesion of leukocytes to endothelial cells and eventually to migration through the expression of various molecules viz, selectins, addresin and integrins. Activation of leukocytes may release numerous mediators including proteases, lipases, lipid metabolites, and free radicals that can be highly toxic to the tissue. Leukocytes not only produce superoxide and hydrogen peroxide through a surface bound enzyme NADPH Oxidase system, but also produce even more toxic halides mediated by myeloperoxidase enzymes. In addition to these free radicals, activated leukocytes are discerned to mobilize iron from ferritin which subsequently may lead to the production of extremely powerful oxidant namely the hydroxyl radical (15). There is potential for a number of positive feed back reactions to transpire due to activation of leukocytes. In this regard Harlan (35) has put forth an interesting idea that following activation of leukocytes and their adhesion to endothelium, a microenvironment is created that would prevent normal protective systems the tissues have through free radical scavengers and protease inhibitors from being effective by excluding these molecules from the region of release. Hence, activation of leukocytes could further lead to enhancement of ischemic damage.

As mentioned earlier, there are experimental studies of several models of cerebral ischemia which have established that leukocytes indeed aggravate the damage caused during ischemia. We have demonstrated that when the number of circulating leukocytes is reduced before inducing transient global cerebral ischemia, the post ischemic neurophysiological recovery was improved when compared to the animals with normal leukocyte count (69). We have also shown (unpublished data) that the infarct size is reduced following global cerebral ischemia in animals made leukopenic prior to ischemia when compared to normopenic controls. Grogaard and coworkers (31) have evinced in a similar ischemic model that leukocytes are involved in the postischemic flow derangements. They were able to demonstrate attenuation of delayed hypoperfusion in certain regions of the brain when antineutrophil serum was administered to a group of animals before inducing ischemia but no improvement in flow when ANS was administered during postischemic reperfuison period. In an air embolus model Dutka and coworkers (21) have also demonstrated improvement of electrophysiological recovery in leukopenic animals. Bednar et al (14) in a thromboembolic model of stroke were able to show improvement in CBF and attenuation of increase in intracranial pressure in neutropenic animals. These results present evidence that the leukocytes may contribute to the exacerbation of cerebral ischemic injury. Further investigation is required to more clearly establish the role of the leukocytes in ischemic and reperfusion injury.

FREE RADICALS

It was Demopolous, Flamm and coworkers who presented the concept of generation of free radicals during ischemia(20,24,25). They correlated the generation of free radicals with cell damage during ischemia. Free radical formation occurs even in normal cells. When the production rate is relatively low, as is the case under normal conditions, the cells have a systematic way of removing free radicals by either enzymatic or nonenzymatic scavenging mechanism. During ischemia and reperfusion the rate of free radical production may overwhelm the scavenging ability of the cells.

There are a number of potential sources for free radical generation in the ischemic brain including mitochondrial respiratory chain, sequences catalyzed by both cyclooxygenase and lipoxygenase, peroxidation of lipid membrane, autooxidation of catecholamines and xanthine oxidase reactions and as mentioned previously leukocytes. Most of the free radicals are highly reactive and readily disappear in the biological system which makes their detection in vivo extremely arduous. In vitro studies have demonstrated the occurrence of lipid peroxidation in brain homogenates (43,56). Also there is indirect evidence to demonstrate the importance of free radical reactions during ischemia. This was based on a decrease in tissue concentration of a naturally occurring free radical scavenger like ascorbic acid in the brain of ischemic animals (24) . In addition there are several studies which report improvement in post ischemic recovery when either enzymatic or non enzymatic free radical scavengers or iron chelators were used. However, during recent years, it has been proved unequivocally through accumulation of conjugated dienes and malonaldehydes that free radicals are generated during ischemia and reperfusion injury (30,71). This offers direct proof for generation of free radicals during cerebral ischemic injury. Nevertheless, there is still a question as to whether free radicals are primarily directly involved in neuronal damage or whether they are predominantly responsible for vascular injury.

OPIOIDS

Opioids are natural compounds which are defined by their specific receptor. Based on the evidence from studies of spinal cord injury where Naloxone, a known narcotic antagonist improved spinal cord flow and neurological function (22,72), it was suggested that Naloxone might also have beneficial effects in the treatment of cerebral ischemia. Ever since the potential beneficial effects of various opioid agonists and antagonists have been examined in different experimental models of cerebral ischemia and in humans with multifarious results. While many studies failed to show any propitious effects of Naloxone (18,27,38,40,41,44,59), an equal number of studies showed improved neurological function (12,23,33,34,39). In addition, evidence for increased B endorphin levels in ischemic brain of animals and CSF of patients have been obtained (26,39,49). We have also provided evidence that opoids have the potential to modulate ischemic damage (70).

The mechanism through which Naloxone may have its beneficial effects is not clearly understood. It is postulated that Naloxone may improve neurological function via a flow related mechanism. However, the results are confounding. There is also a question whether Naloxone has its ameliorating effects via mu (endorphin) opioid receptor because the dose at which the beneficial effects of Naloxone is evinced is considered to be too high for mu receptor antagonizing effects. At such high doses, Naloxone is believed to have or possess antagonistic effects on Kappa (dynorphin) receptors. Of late, there is some evidence that high doses of Naloxone may also antagonize excitatory amino acids (42).

The results of Kappa receptor agonist and antagonist drugs are even more confounding. Both Kappa agonists (13,33,68) and antagonists (2) have exhibited protective effects in animal models of cerebral ischemia. It was presumed that the Kappa receptor selective agonist used in those studies appeared to have action on the nonopioid systems. It is even more befogging as activation of kappa receptors has been found to inhibit calcium uptake and subsequent excitatory amino acid release (16).

Based on these ambivalent results, it could be conjectured that perhaps several opioid actions which are mutually active and/or counteractive are involved in the pathophysiology of cerebral ischemia. Some of these mechanisms might be beneficial and others may be deleterious to the outcome following cerebral ischemia. However, it is beyond dispute that opioids modulate the pathophysiology of cerebral ischemic injury.

EXCITATORY AMINO ACIDS

The possible role of excitatory neurotransmitters in cerebral ischemia has recently received a lot of attention. Cerebral ischemia causes an increased release and a decreased reuptake of the excitatory neurotransmitters glutamate and aspartate. This results in an increased level of these excitatory aminoacids in the extracellular space which will lead to excitation of adjacent neurons and further depletion of energy stores. This positive feed back action is believed to cause two types of damage (osmolytic and calcium related) based on the time course and ionic conductance (62). The first component of damage is based on the activation of kainate and AMPA receptors which result in an increase in the conductance of sodium. Secondarily to increased sodium influx, chloride and water will enter. Consequently cell swelling will occur (Osmolytic damage). The second component of damage is due to the activation of NMDA receptors resulting in increased calcium influx which is characterized by delayed neuronal injury. Hitherto, various competitive and noncompetitive NMDA antagonists were tested in different types of cerebral ischemic models with varying results. Whereas most of the studies showed beneficial effects of NMDA antagonists when administered systemically (29,45,51,66), a few studies failed to evince any positive effects. Some of the beneficial effects reported appeared to be secondary to the hypothermic effect of the blocker. The potential role of these agents in cerebral protection remains to be clarified.

Lately, a newer non-NMDA antagonist NBQX (AMPA receptor blocker) was found to be a neuroprotectant in a global ischemic model, even when administered 2 hrs after the ischemic insult (58). Even though the exact mechanism of action of this drug is not clearly understood, it is thought that its neuroprotective effect is not exerted via a non-specific sedative or hypothermic effect.

It is beyond the scope of this chapter to deal with pharmacological attenuation of excitatory damage; however, Table 1,2,3, and 4 list NMDA receptor agonists and antagonists, competitive NMDA antagonists with their relative anticonvulsant potencies, non-competitive NMDA antagonists and their potencies, and non-NMDA antagonists respectively.

CONCLUSION

The pathophysiological mechanisms of cerebral ischemia and reperfusion injury is quite complicated and confounding because of the multitude of factors which are interacting and/or opposing to one another. This offers a definite challenge for the clinicians in treating ischemic injury of the brain. Finally, these newfangled mechanisms of pathogenesis of cerebral ischemic damage, need not exclude conventional therapies used hitherto. However, it is intended to provide newer insights into novel therapeutic directives to include manipulation of various different systems and to apportion a "cocktail version" with a synergistic effect.

REFERENCES

1.　　Ames III, A., B.S. Gurian, Effects of glucose and oxygen deprivation on function of isolated mammalian retina. *J. Neurophysiol.* 26:617-634, 1963.

2.　　Andrews, B.T., T.K. Mcintosh, M.F. Gonzales, P.R. Neinstein, and A.J. Faden, Levels of endogenous opiods and effects of an opiate antagonist during regional cerebral ischemia in rats. *J. Pharmacol Experimental Therapeutics.* 247(3): 1248-1254, 1988.

3.　　Astrup, J., B.K. Siesjo, and L. Symon, Thresholds in cerebral ischemia - the ischemic penumbra. *Stroke.* 12:723-725, 1981.

4.　　Astrup, J., L. Symon, N.M. Branston, and N.A. Lassen, Cortical evoked potential and extracellular K^+ and H^+ at critical levels of brain ischemia. *Stroke.* 8:51-57, 1977.

5.　　Barber, A.A. and F. Bernheim, Lipid peroxidation: Its measurement, occurrence and significance in animal tissues. *Adv. Gerontol. Res 2:* 355-403, 1967.

6.　　Baron, J.C. The study of cerebral circulation using positron emission tomography. *Minerva. Med* .79:651-653, 1988.

7.　　Baron, J.C., M.G. Bousser, D. Comar, D. Rougemont, P. Lebrun Grandie, and P. Castaigne, Positron emission tomography in the physiopathological study of cerebral ischemia in man. *Presse Med.* 12:3066-3072, 1983.

8.　　Baron, J.C. , M.G. Bousser, D. Comar, F. Soussaline and P. Castaigne, Noninvasive tomographic study of cerebral blood flow and oxygen metabolism in vivo. Potentials, limitations, and clinical applications in cerebral ischemic disorders. *Eur. Neurol.* 20:273-284, 1981.

9.   Baron, J.C., Bousser, M.G., Rey A., Guillard, A., Comar, D. and Castaigne, P. Reversal of focal "misery-perfusion syndrome" by extra-intracranial arterial bypass in hemodynamic cerebral ischemia. A case study with 150 positron emission tomography. *Stroke.* 12:454-459, 1981.

10.   Baron, J.C., R. D'Antona, M. Serdaru, P. Pantano, M.G. Bousser, and Y. Samson. Cortical hypometabolism after a thalamic lesion in man: positron tomography study. *Rev. Neurol.* 142:465-474, 1986.

11.   Baron, J.C., D. Rougemont, F. Soussaline, F., et al.: Local interrelationships of cerebral oxygen consumption and glucose utilization in normal subjects and in ischemic stroke patients: A positron tomography study. *J Cereb Blood Flow Metab* .4:140-149, 1984.

12.   Baskin, D.S., and Y. Hosobuchi, Naloxone reversal of ischaemic neurologic deficits in man. *Lancet* : 2: 272-275, 1981.

13.   Baskin, D.S., H. Kuroda, Y. Hosobuchi , and N.M. Lee, Treatment of Stroke with opiate antagonists- Effects of enogenous antagonists and dynorphin 1-13. *Neuropeptides* 5:307-310, 1985.

14.   Bednar, M.M., S. Raymond, T. McAuliffe, P.A. Lodge, and C.E Gross, The role of neutrophils and platelets in a rabbit model of thromboembolic *Stroke.* 22:44-50, 1991.

15.   Biemond, P., H.G. Van Eijk, A.J.G. Seaak, and J.F. Koster, Iron mobilization from ferritin by superoxide derived from stimulated polymorphonuclear leukocytes: Possible mechanisms in inflammation diseases. *J. Clin. Invest*: 73, 1576-1579, 1984.

16.   Bradford H.F., J.M. Crowder, and E.J. White, Inhibitory actions of opioid compounds on calcium fluxes and neurotransmitter release from mammalian cerebral cortical slices. *Br. J. Pharmocol* .88:87-93, 1986.

17.   Branston, N.M., A.J. Stong, and L. Symon, Extracellular potassium activity, evoked potential and tissue blood flow. Relationships during progressive ischaemia in baboon cerebral cortex. *J. Neurol Sci.* 32:305-321, 1977.

18.   CapdeVille, C., D. Pruneau, M. Allin, M. Plotkine, & R.G. Boulu, Does naloxone reverse the neurologic deficit induced by global cerebral ischemia in rats? *J. CBF. Metab* 3(Suppl 1):532-533, 1983.

19.   Choi, D.W., H. Monyer, R.G. Giffard, M.P. Goldberg, and C.W. Christine, Acute brain injury, NMDA receptors, and hydrogen ions: Observations in cortical cell cultures. *Adv. Exp. Med. Biol.* 268:501-504, 1990.

20.   Demopoulos, H., E. Flamm, M. Seligmann, R. Power, D. Pietronigro, J. Ransohoff, Molecular pathology of lipids in CNS membranes In: *Oxygen and Physiological Function* (Jobsin F.F. ed). pp 491-508. Dallas, Texas. 1977.

21.   Dutka, A., P. Kochanek, J. Hallenbeck, Influence of granulocytopenia on canine cerebral ischemia induced by air embolism. *Stroke* 20: 390 - 395, 1990.

22.   Faden, A.J., T.P. Jacobs, and J.W. Holaday,   Opiate antagonist improves neurological recovery after spinal injury. *Science*. 211:493 - 494, 1981.

23.   Faden, A.J., J.M. Hallenbeck, and C.Q. Brown, Treatment of experimental stroke: comparison of naloxone and thyrotropin releasing hormone. *Neurology* 32: 1083-1087, 1982.

24.   Flamm, E.S., H.B. Demopoulous,M.L. Seligmann,P.G. Poser, J. Ronsohoff, Free radicals in cerebral ischemia. *Stroke* 9: 445-447, 1978.

25.   Flamm, E.S., H.B. Demopoulos, H.L. Seligman, J. Ransohoff, Possible molecular mechanisms of barbiturate - mediated protection in regional cerebral ischemia. *Acta Neurol. Scand. (Suppl 64)* 56:150-151, 1977.

26.   Furui, T., K. Satoh, Y. Asano, S. Shimosawa, M. Hasuo, and T.L. Yaksh, Increase of β-endorphin levels in cerebral infarction. *J. Neurosurg* 61:748 - 751, 1984.

27.   Gaines, C., D.G. Nehls, D.M. Suess, J.D. Waggener, and R.M. Crowell, R.M.: Effect of naloxone on experimental stroke in awake monkeys. *Neurosurgery*. 14:308-314, 1984.

28.   Garcia, J.H.: Experimental ischemic stroke: A review. *Stroke*. 15: 5 -14, 1984.

29.   Gill, R., A.C. Foster, and G.N., Systemic administration of MK-801 protects against ischemia-induced hippocampal neurodegeneration in the gerbil. *J. Neurosci.* 7:3343-3349, 1987.

30.   Ginsberg, M.D., B.D. Watson, S. Yoshida, R. Busto, K. Abe, W.J. Goldberg, and P. Scheinberg, Aspects of tissue injury in cerebral ischemia. In : Cerbro vascular diseases. pp. 237-250, (M. Reivich and H.J. Hurtig (ed.s) *Raven Press*, New York, 1983.

31. Grogaard, B., L. Schurer, B. Gerdin,   and K.E. Arfors, Delayed hypoperfusion after incomplete forebrain ischemia in the rat. The role of polymorphonuclear leukocytes. *J. Cereb Blood Flow Metab* . 9:500-505, 1989.

32.   Grotta, J.C., C.M. Picone, P.T. Ostrow, et al. CGS-19755, A competitive NMDA receptor antagonist, reduces calcium-calmodulin binding and improves outcome after global cerebral ischemia. *Ann. Neurol.* 27:612-619, 1990.

33.   Handa, N., M. Matsumoto, K. Kitagawa, A. Uehara, S. Ogawa, H. Wtani, S. Yoneda, K. Kimura, and T. Kamada, Levallorphan and dynorphin improve motor dysfunction in mongolian gerbils with unilateral carotid occlusion: The first application of the inclined plane method in the experimental ischemia. *Life Sci.* 42: 1825 - 1831, 1988.

34.   Handa, N., M. Matsumoto, M. Nakamura, S. Yoneda, K. Kimura, Y. Sugitani, K Tanaka, T. Takano, and T. Kamada, Reversal of neurological deficits by Levallorphan in patients with acute ischemic stroke. *J. CBF Metab* 5: 469-472, 1985.

35.   Harlan, J.M.: Leukocyte endothelial interactions. *Blood.* 65:513-525, 1985

36.   Harris, R.J., L. Symon, N.M. Branston, and M. Bayhan, Changes in extracellular calcium activity in cerebral ischaemia. *J. Cereb. Blood Flow Metab.* 1:203-209, 1981.

37.   Heiss, W.D. Therapy of cerebral ischaemia. *Z.Kardiol.* 76 Suppl 4:87-98, 1987.

38.   Holaday, J.W. and R.J. D'Amato, Nalaxone or TRH fails to improve neurologic deficits in gerbil models of "Stroke." *Life Sci.* 31: 385-392, 1982.

39.   Hosobuchi, Y., D.S. Baskin, and S.K. Woo, Reversal of induced ischemic neurologic deficit in gerbils by the opiate antagonist naloxone. *Science* 215: 69-71, 1982.

40.   Hubbard, J.L. and T.M. Sundt, Failure of naloxone to affect focal incomplete cerebral ischemia and collateral blood flow in cats. *J. Neurosurgery.* 59:237-244, 1983.

41.   Kastin, A.J., C. Nissen, and R.D. Olson, Failure of MIF. 1 or naloxone to reverse ischemic - induced neurologic deficits in gerbils. *Pharmacol Biochem and Behau* .17: 1083 - 1085, 1982.

42.   Kim, J.P., M.P. Goldberg, and D.W. Choi, High concentrations of Naloxone attenuate NMDA receptor mediated neurotoxicity. *Eur J. Pharmocol.* 138:133-136, 1987.

43.   Kogure, K., H. Arai, K. Abe, and M. Nakamo, Free radical damage of the brain following ischemia. *Progress in Brain Research.* 63: 237-259, 1985.

44.   Levy, R.M., M. Stryker, and Y. Hosobuchi, Studies of nuclear magnetic resonance imaging and regional cerebral glucose metabolism in acute cerebral ischemia Possible mechanism of opiate antagonist therapeutic activity. *Life Sci.* 33: 763-768, 1983.

45.   McDonald, J.N., F.S. Silverstein, M.V. Johnston, MK-801 protects the neonatal brain from hypoxic-ischemic damage. *Eur. J. Pharmacol.* 140:359-361, 1987.

46.   Meldrum, B. Possible therapeutic applications of antagonists of excitatory amino acid neurotransmitters. *Clin Sci.* 68:113-122, 1985.

47.   Myers, R.E., G.S. Kopf, and D.M. Mirvis, Hemodynamic response to profound hypoxia in intact rhesus monkeys. *Stroke.* 11:389-393, 1980.

48.   Myers, R.E. and S. Yamaguchi, Nervous system effects of cardiac arrest in monkeys. Preservation of vision. *Arch Neurol* 34:65-74, 1977.

49.   Nappi, G., F. Facchinetti, G. Bono, F. Petraglia, E. Sinforiani, A.R. and Genazzani, CSF and plasma levels of pro-opiomelanocortin related peptides in reversible ischemic attacks and strokes. *J. Neurol Neurosurg Psychiatry* 49: 17-21, 1986.

50.   Nowycky, M.C., A.P. Fox, R.W. Tsien, Three types of neuronal calcium channel with different calcium agonist sensitivity *Nature (London)* 316:440-443, 1985.

51.   Ozyurt, E., D.I. Graham, G.N. Woodruff, and J. McCulloch, Protective effect of the glutamate antagonist, MK-801 in focal cerebral ischemia in the cat. *J. CBF. Metab* 8:138-143, 1988.

52.   Petito, C.K., W.A. Pulsinelli, G. Jacobson, Edema and vascular permeability in cerebral ischemia: comparison between ischemic neuronal damage and infarction. *J. Neuropathol. Exp. Neurol.* 41: 423 - 437, 1982.

53.   Plum, F.: What causes infarction in ischemic brain? The Robert Wartenberg Lecture. *Neurology* 33: 222 - 233 , 1983.

54.   Pulsinelli, W.A., D.E. Levy, B. Sigsbee, P. Scherer and F. Plum, Increased damage after ischemic stroke in patients with hyperglycemia with or without established diabetes mellitus. *Am. J. Med.* 74:540-544, 1983.

55.   Pulsinelli, W.A., S. Waldman, D. Rawlinson, and F. Plum, Moderate hyperglycemia augments ischemic brain damage: a neuropathologic study in the rat. *Neurology.* 32:1239-1246, 1982

56.   Rehncrona, S., J. Folbergrova, D.S. Smith, and B.K. Siesjo, Influence of complete and pronounced incomplete cerebral ischemia and subsequent recirculation on cortical concentrations of oxidized and reduced glutathione in the rat. *J. Neurochem* 34 (3) : 477 - 486, 1980.

57.   Rehncrona, S., E.O. Nielsen, H. Hauge , B.K. Siesjo, Enhancement of iron - catalyzed free radical formation by acidosis in brain homogenates: difference in effect by lactid acid and CO_2. *J. Cereb Blood Flow Metab* 9:65-70, 1989.

58.   Sheardown, M.J., E.O. Nielsen, A.J. Hansen, P. Jacobsen, and T. Honore, 2-3-dihydroxy-6-nitro-7-sulfamoyl-benzo(F)quinoxaline:A neuroprotectant for cerebral ischemia. *Science* 247:571-574, 1990.

59.   Shigeno, T., G.M. Teasdle, D. Kirkhan, D. Mendelow, D.J. Graham, and J. McCulloch, Effect of naloxone on cerebral glucose metabolism in normal rats and rats with focal cerebral ischemia. *J. CBF Metab. 3(Suppl 1)*: 528-529, 1983.

60.   Siesjo, B.K.: Cell damage in the brain: A speculative synthesis. *J. Cereb. Blood Flow. Metab.* 1: 155-185, 1981.

61.   Siesjo, B.K.: Cerebral circulation and metabolism. *J. Neurosurgery* 60: 883 - , 1984.

62.   Siesjo, B.K.: Mechanisms of ischemic brain damage. *Crit Care Med.* 16(10) : 954-964, 1988.

63.   Siesjo, B.K., G. Bendek, T. Koide, E. Westerberg, and T. Wieloch, Influence of acidosis on lipid peroxidation in brain tissues in vitro. *J. Cereb Blood Flow Metab.* 5:253-258, 1985.

64.   Siesjo, B.K. and F. Bengsten, Calcium fluxes, calcium antagonists and calcium related pathology in brain ischemia, hypoglycemia and spreading depression: a unifying hypothesis. *J. Cereb Blood Flow Metab* 9:127-140, 1989.

65.   Simon, R.P., J.H. Swan, T. Griffiths, and B.S. Meldrum, Blockade of N-methyl-D-asparate receptors may protect against ischemic damage in the brain. Science 226:850-852, 1984.

66.   Simon, R.P., J.W. Schmidley, B.S. Meldrum, J.H. Swan, and A.G. Chapman, Excitotoxic mechanisms in hypoglycaemic hippocampal injury. Neuropathol. Appl. Neurobiol. 12:567-576, 1986.

67.   Smith, M.L., R.N. Auer, B.K. Siesjo, The density and distribution of ischemic brain injury in the rat following two to ten minutes of forebrain ischemia. *Acta Neuropathol* 64:319. 1984.

68.   Tang, A.H.: Protection from cerebral ischemia by U-50,488E, a specific kappa opiod analgesic. *Life Sci.* 37:1475-1482, 1985.

69.   Vasthare, U.S., L.A. Heinel, R.H. Rossenwasser, and R.F. Tuma, Leukocyte involvement in cerebral ischemia and reperfusion injury. *Surg. Neurol.* 33: 261-265, 1990.

70.   Vasthare, U.S., S. Rubin, H.A. Riina, R.H. Rosenwasser, C. Carlsson, and R.F. Tuma, Effect of fentanyl on the electrophysiological recovery following incomplete global cerebral ischemia. *Drug Develop Res* 23: 227-232, 1991.

71.   Wei, E.P., H.A. Kontos, W.D. Dietrich, et al: Inhibition by free radical scavengers and by cyclooxygenase inhibitors of pial arteriolar abnormalities from concussive brain injury in cats. *Circ Res :* 48:95 - 1981.

72.   Young, W., E.S. Flamm, H.B. Demopoulos, J.J. Tomasula, and V. Decrescito, Effect of naloxone on post traumatic ischemia in experimental spinal contusion. *J. Neurosurgery* 55L 209-219, 1981.

3

HEMODYNAMIC AND BIOCHEMICAL IMPLICATIONS OF VASCULAR CELLS IN CEREBRAL ISCHEMIA/REPERFUSION: FUTURE DIRECTIONS FOR TREATMENT

Michelle C. Mazzoni[*] and Karl-E. Arfors

The La Jolla Institute for Experimental Medicine
La Jolla, CA 92037

and

*Department of AMES-Bioengineering
University of California, La Jolla, CA 92093

INTRODUCTION

Hypoxic and ischemic insults to nervous and brain tissue are inflicted to varying degrees by vascular occlusions, trauma to the central nervous system (CNS), and global ischemia (e.g., hemorrhage). In these low-flow and oxygen-deprived states, a variety of pathophysiological changes take place which are dependent on the severity and duration of the insult. For example, when cerebral blood flow (CBF) is decreased to one-third of its normal level, there is an inhibition of evoked synaptic responses. A further flow reduction to one-fifth or less of normal greatly impairs ATP synthesis with the rapid depletion of tissue energy stores. If this condition persists beyond a few minutes, the cell membrane ion pumps, which demand a ceaseless supply of ATP, can no longer compensate to keep in balance the ion influx via ion channels, exchangers, and leaks. Cell membrane depolarization ensues with an attendant increase in intracellular calcium and sodium and extracellular potassium. Ischemic insults with such tissue cell membrane depolarization are thought to trigger events that can lead to neuronal damage (Siesjo et al., 1988).

Many cellular processes are activated during CNS ischemia. Those which are possibly involved in neuronal injury can be classified into the following areas:

1. Ion (hydrogen, calcium, sodium) transport and water shifts across the cell membrane.
2. Transmitter release and agonist-receptor interactions.
3. Arachidonic acid release and oxygen-free radical formation.
4. Changes in the intracellular signalling system (calcium ions, phospholipid turnover).
5. Altered protein chemistry, including changes in gene expressions and protein modification (phosphorylation, proteolysis) (Wieloch, 1990).

Discussions pertaining to these neurochemical processes are prevalent in the literature. Much of the findings have evolved from studies in *in vitro* cell systems, however, an increasing number of *in vivo* models are being developed to examine the impact of cellular dysfunction on brain injury, recovery, and survival in ischemia/hypoxia and trauma.

Reperfusion has been found to exacerbate ischemic injury in the brain, as well as most other organs, suggesting a common denominator for the response irrespective of the type of tissue cell. A hemodynamic genesis could be suspected based on the observation that microcirculatory blood flow remains depressed and becomes maldistributed with the return of supply flow to the tissue, the so-called "slow" or "no-reflow" phenomenon. In fact, no-reflow was first described in the brain by Ames and coworkers in 1968. Besides delivering oxygen to the tissue via the red blood cells (RBCs), the blood circulates other chemical substances (e.g., metabolic byproducts) and cells including white blood cells (WBCs) and platelets through the endothelial cell (EC)-lined vessels. Thus, it may be some change in the blood composition or events occurring at the endothelial interface between blood and tissue cells, in addition to a deficient level of blood flow, which are factors in the development of no-reflow.

In this chapter, a different approach to thinking about cerebral ischemia/reperfusion is presented which focuses on the extracellular contribution to neuronal cell derangement, as opposed to the intracellular mechanisms mentioned above. Specifically discussed are the hemodynamic and biochemical roles of the vascular cells, of interest here are capillary endothelium and WBCs. Two novel and exciting therapeutic methods aimed directly at these vascular cells, hyperosmotic fluid resuscitation and monoclonal antibody therapy, are introduced. The conceptual framework is based on results from *in vitro* and *in vivo* studies using various organs and species. This broad spectrum of data affords a generalized description of the ischemia/reperfusion problem, with answers specific for the brain updated as knowledge from suitable models is acquired.

HEMODYNAMIC FACTORS IN ISCHEMIA/REPERFUSION

BLOOD FLOW REDUCTION

In situations of reduced systemic arterial pressure (e.g., hemorrhagic shock), autoregulation via local regulatory mechanisms and reflexes in the brain maintains a constant CBF. Thus, decreases in CBF are usually localized phenomenon, caused by vessel obstruction or aneurysm (e.g., stroke) or external compression (e.g., edema from traumatic injury) which compromises flow to distal brain regions. This condition may be aggravated by concomitant hypotension resulting from severe and extended trauma. Because the brain can only tolerate flow deprivation for a few minutes before permanent cell damage occurs, the rapid and sufficient restoration of CBF after an ischemic episode is an important problem in clinical medicine. Understanding the pathophysiology of ischemia/reperfusion in the brain is still ongoing, with considerable insight provided from experimental models in the brain as well as other organs.

Bednar et al. (1991) in a rabbit model of thromboembolic stroke drastically reduced CBF with a synergistic combination of systemic (hypotension) and local flow reductions (embolization). Besides CBF, intracranial pressure (ICP) was measured after a 45 minute hypotensive period and in the time following the restoration of baseline blood pressure, along with the cerebral infarct size at the end of this reperfusion period. Arterial pH and blood gases were maintained throughout the experiment. Three groups of animals were studied. In two groups, either the neutrophils or platelets were selectively removed from the blood circulation. The third (control) group had unaltered neutrophil and platelet counts.

A key finding of the study was that in the neutropenic group with the return of supply blood pressure, CBF was restored significantly better as compared to the control group, although not to baseline values, and the otherwise two-fold increase in ICP was prevented. The results for the platelet-free group were intermediate between the neutropenic and control groups. To note is that in all groups, there was a pronounced incomplete recovery of CBF. This result reaffirms earlier reported evidence for the "no-reflow" or "slow-reflow" phenomenon in the brain as well as many other organs in the body on reperfusion following a prolonged ischemic insult, due to either total or incomplete flow occlusion.

With arterial blood pressure restored, the persistent reduction in CBF could be attributed to either a decrease in the net pressure gradient across the cerebral blood vessels ($\Delta P = P_{art} - P_{ven}$) or an increase in the resistance to flow (R) in these vessels. According to Poiseuille's Law:

$$CBF = \Delta P / R \qquad (1)$$

This relationship is a gross simplification of the actual hemodynamics, but it facilitates thinking on the cause of the no-reflow observation. It is conceivable that P_{ven} is increased by excessive neutrophil sticking in the postcapillary venules, a frequent post-ischemia observation, but CBF was found to remain depressed even when these WBCs were removed. This leaves R, therefore, as a primary hemodynamic factor contributing to the insufficient flow recovery on reperfusion.

INCREASES IN BLOOD VESSEL RESISTANCE

The resistance in equation (1) represents that of an entire organ, of interest here is the brain. The cerebral arteries, veins, and capillaries are arranged in series with one another, therefore, the corresponding expression for R can be written analogous to electrical circuit theory as

$$R = R_{art} + R_{ven} + R_{cap} \qquad (2)$$

The individual members of each type of vessel lie in parallel with one another. For example, in the capillary network the spanning resistance R_{cap} is a function of each individual capillary resistance. Assuming a uniform capillary bed with no cross-connections, R_{cap} can be expressed as

$$1 / R_{cap} = N / R_p \qquad (3)$$

where N is the number of parallel capillaries (R_p). Continuing further, the resistance in a single blood vessel can be represented by the hydraulic resistance in a cylindrical tube according to the equation

$$R = k \, \eta \, 1 / r^4 \qquad (4)$$

where k is a proportionality constant, η is blood viscosity, 1 is vessel length, and r is the vessel radius. This relation assumes the flow is steady and the fluid is homogeneous (Newtonian). In the circulation, the length of any given vessel is virtually constant. The viscosity, which for a given size vessel is a function of the particulate nature of the blood, does not normally vary appreciably. In pathological or hemodiluted states, however, the viscosity could change and contribute to resistance changes. But the main alterations in resistance are produced, physiologically and pathophysiologically, by virtue of the strong dependence on changes in vessel radius.

The majority of organ resistance, approximately 75%, resides in the arterial system with the veins and capillaries each adding about 10% and 15%, respectively. Arterioles are capable of large resistance fluctuations via changes in caliber so vasoconstriction could increase resistance and decrease reflow. And even venules clogged by RBC stasis and adherent WBCs could elevate organ resistance and further limit flow. But the no-reflow phenomenon has been attributed to events prevailing at the capillary level. In a skeletal muscle model of pressure-induced total ischemia (four hours), the number of perfused capillaries 24 hours after blood reperfusion was found to be 50% of the number prior to ischemia (Menger et al., 1988). After the low-flow ischemia produced by hemorrhagic shock (two hours), reperfusion with enough blood or iso-osmotic fluids to restore systemic circulatory function led to a persistent sluggish and maldistributed capillary network flow in skeletal muscle with many capillaries remaining nonperfused after two hours (Amundson et al., 1980b). These studies and others demonstrate that insufficient microcirculatory reflow after reperfusion is the manifestation of abnormalities in capillary distribution. Capillary flow dysfunction is already evident during low-flow ischemia (Amundson et al., 1980a). Reduced and maldistributed flow has serious consequences in terms of vital nutrient and metabolite diffusional exchange between blood and tissue.

Diminished flow and the loss of a regular intermittent perfusion pattern as observed in skeletal muscle capillaries during low-flow ischemia and reperfusion suggests that the hydraulic resistances in and among capillaries are exaggerated. Preferentially high-resistance capillaries become even higher as compared to adjacent capillaries with the result that they receive little if any flow, especially in combination with low perfusion pressures. The causes postulated for the increase and widened dispersion in resistances include RBC aggregation, platelet and WBC trapping, and swelling of tissue and capillary ECs (Lewis, 1984). Each possible cause has its proponents based on a variety of experimental models. Specifically for the brain, the precise causes are unknown.

ENDOTHELIAL CELL SWELLING - CAPILLARY NARROWING AND WHITE BLOOD CELL PLUGGING

The reflow response during reperfusion after an incomplete (low-flow) ischemia in the brain is improved, but not restored to baseline values, by the removal of circulating WBCs (Bednar et al., 1991; GrRgaard et al., 1989) or platelets (Bednar et al., 1991). Thus, additional mechanisms must be operative to account for impaired cerebral reperfusion. There is considerable evidence for cell swelling in low-flow and total ischemia, including skeletal muscle cell edema after hemorrhagic shock (Nakayama et al., 1985; Shires et al., 1972) and EC edema in the capillaries of totally ischemic skeletal muscle (Gidlof et al., 1982, 1987), heart (Kloner et al., 1974), and kidney (Flores et al., 1972; Frega et al., 1976). And swelling may actually be exacerbated by blood reflow, since histological examination of totally ischemic organs minutes after reperfusion revealed an even higher incidence of edematous ECs (Gidlof et al., 1982, 1987; Kloner et al., 1974).

Intravital microscopy studies of the rabbit tenuissimus muscle have shown that during hemorrhagic shock, the capillaries narrow as a result of EC swelling (Mazzoni et al., 1989). This is the first documentation of capillary EC edema in a low-flow ischemia. The swollen cells encroach on the capillary lumen and decrease the diameter for flow as shown in Figure 1. The corresponding single vessel resistance increase is also given assuming a uniform capillary narrowing as described by Equation 4. The significance of the marked increase in single capillary resistance is two-fold. First, variations in the degree of narrowing between neighboring capillaries could exaggerate the relative resistances and redistribute flow by shunting blood through lower resistance capillaries, with some capillaries continuously deprived of flow. Secondly, it may contribute to the trapping of WBCs, which are larger and much stiffer than RBCs. WBCs have been observed in nonperfused capillaries during hemorrhagic shock (Amundson et al., 1980a), and with blood reperfusion after shock (Amundson et al., 1980b; Bagge et al., 1980; Barroso-Aranda et al., 1988) and organ ischemia (Engler et al., 1983).

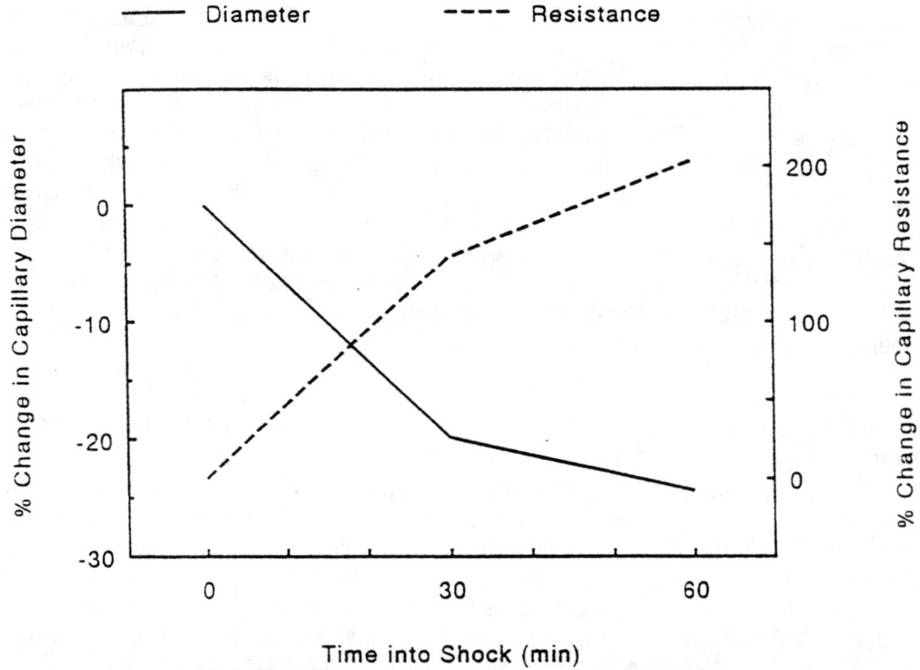

Figure 1: The percent decrease in capillary diameter due to EC swelling during the low-flow ischemia of hemorrhagic shock (40% bleed of total blood volume). Corresponding to the capillary narrowing of almost 25% after one hour of shock is a dramatic increase in the hydraulic resistance to flow. This resistance increase may play a role in the no-reflow phenomenon.

The resistance across the capillary network will be less than that of any single vessel (Equation 3), however, its relative increase when the capillaries narrow can be much greater. Furthermore, network resistance is elevated if N decreases because of nonperfused capillaries or ones transiently or irreversibly plugged with WBCs. If in a network of 30 capillaries (Warnke and Skalak, 1990), each had a 24% diameter reduction and corresponding 200% resistance increase (Figure 1) which caused flow to cease in half of them, the resistance of the network would increase by 500%! The actual extent of EC swelling which produces the capillary narrowing is probably much less than has been assumed for this calculation, but its impact is clearly illustrated. And even though the capillaries normally contribute only 15% to organ resistance, this value rises to 47% for a 500% increase in network resistance (Equation 2). With the restoration of blood pressure, the overall 60% increase in organ resistance would account for a significant reduction in blood flow (Equation 1).

FLUID RESUSCITATION - HYPEROSMOTIC FLUIDS

Capillaries narrowed by swollen endothelium with elevated resistances pose a physical hindrance to reflow. As previously described, the no-reflow phenomenon has been well-documented for reperfusion with blood or iso-osmotic fluids. These fluids adequately restore systemic circulatory parameters, but their ineffectiveness to reinstate microcirculatory flow may be in that they do not reverse the EC swelling. Because of their theoretical attractiveness in shrinking swollen cells, hyperosmotic solutions (2,400 mosm/L) have been tried as a resuscitation fluid with the specific and unique aim to treat narrowed capillaries. It was found that a bolus infusion of 7.5% NaCl/6% dextran 70 (HSD) fully reinstated capillary flow and rectified diameter (Mazzoni et al., 1990). The diameter recovery is shown in Figure 2 along with the result that the isotonic fluid Ringer's lactate (RL) was ineffectual in restoring diameter. The reopening of narrowed capillaries would explain why, in contrast to conventional reperfusion with blood or iso-osmotic fluids, hyperosmotic solutions given after hemorrhagic shock have been found to restore microcirculatory flow (Kreimeier and Messmer, 1987). We attribute the favorable response largely to the osmotic redraw of water from swollen ECs.

On a larger scale, the osmotic mechanism of action of hypertonic saline/dextran solutions causes a rapid redistribution of water from the cells and interstitium into the plasma, thereby restoring circulating blood volume (Mazzoni et al., 1988). Small infusion volumes of these innovative solutions have been judged effective as a fluid therapy for hypovolemic hemorrhage in both experimental (Maningas et al., 1986; Smith et al., 1985) and clinical settings (Holcroft et al., 1987; Maningas et al., 1989). There have been no reports (experimental or clinical) of adverse microvascular permeability effects owing directly to hyperosmotic resuscitation. In fact, peripheral edema is often found to be minimized and also studies have shown that there may be benefit for trauma patients with neurological injury. ICP was lowered with hypertonic saline infusions (3% or 7.5%) as compared to resuscitation with RL, dextran 40 (10%), or normal saline after a hypotensive shock period (Gunnar et al., 1986; Prough et al., 1985), even with a simulated head injury (Gunnar et al., 1988).

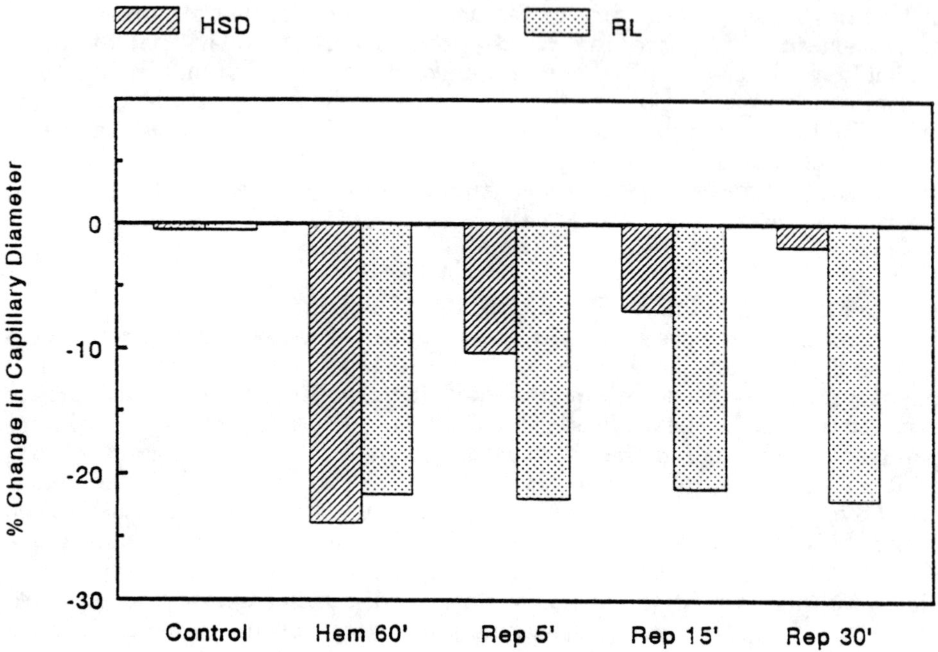

Figure 2: Percent changes in capillary diameters after shock (Hem) and reperfusion (Rep) with a bolus infusion of either 7.5% NaCl/6% dextran 70 (HSD, dose equal to one-seventh of the shed blood volume) or Ringer's lactate (RL, dose equal to the shed blood volume). HSD completely restored capillary diameter 30 minutes after infusion, but RL was ineffective.

BIOCHEMICAL FACTORS IN ISCHEMIA/REPERFUSION

TISSUE ACIDOSIS

During an ischemic insult, tissue acidosis develops from an enhanced lactic acid formation as cells must shift from aerobic to anaerobic metabolism. Figure 3 shows the various ion pathways and chemical process involved in cellular acidification. Intracellular H^+ concentration increases which then activates pH regulatory Na^+/H^+ exchange (Cala et al., 1988; Frelin et al., 1987). The electroneutral Na^+/H^+ antiport exchanges intracellular H^+ for extracellular Na^+ with an attendant net influx of Cl^+, assuming competent Cl^+/HCO_3^- exchange. Unless the excess Na^+ is removed, the solute concentration inside the cell increases and edema from osmotically obliged water ensues. The increased cellular Na^+ content could also conceivably result from an enhanced inward movement of Na^+ down its concentration gradient via Na^+ channels. It has been shown, however, that select inhibition of the Na^+/H^+ exchanger and not the Na^+ channel with infusion of the drug amiloride and its analogs prior to hemorrhage prevents the otherwise shock-induced swelling of capillary ECs (Mazzoni et al., 1992).

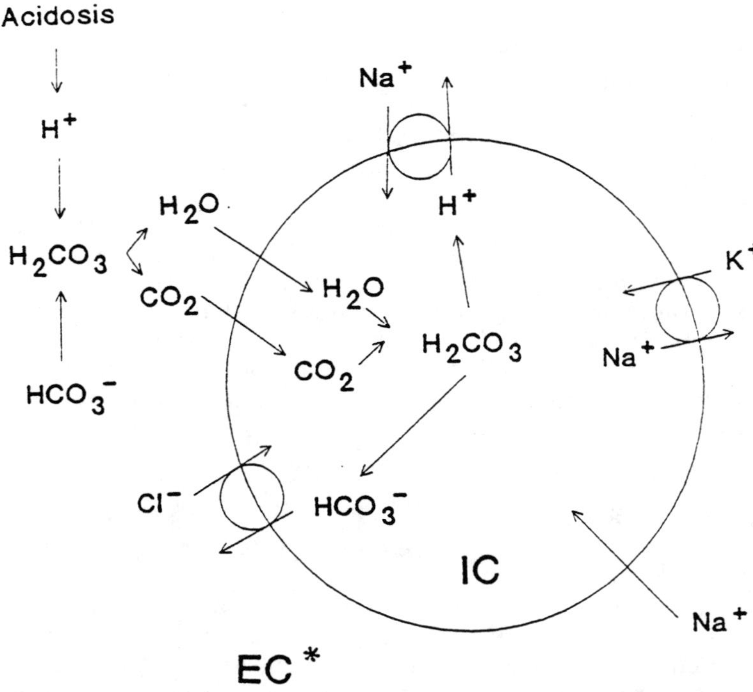

Figure 3: Ion pathways and biochemical processes which may play a role in ischemic cell swelling via tissue acidosis. In extracellular acidosis, H^+ ions accumulate in the extracellular space (EC*) which could then be buffered by bicarbonate (HCO_3^-) resulting in the formation of carbonic acid (H_2CO_3) and subsequent dissociation into carbon dioxide (CO_2) and water (H_2O). After diffusing into the cell, CO_2 recombines with water again to form H_2CO_3 which then decays into H^+ and HCO_3^-. Now the H^+ is intracellular (IC) and like direct intracellular acidification, the H^+ is eliminated by Na^+/H^+ exchange with concomitant Cl^-/HCO_3^- exchange. The Na^+/K^+ pump and passive Na^+ conductance via channels do not appear to have primary roles in hypoxic cell swelling.

In the brain, even cells themselves not hypoxic can be exposed to an increased H+ milieu because the brain is a closed compartment and hypoxic cells extrude H+ into the extracellular space. Cell swelling has been shown for C6 glial cells (Jakubovicz and Klip, 1989) on intracellular acidification, and C6 glioma/glial cells (Jakubovicz et al., 1987; Jakubovicz and Klip, 1989; Kempski et al., 1988) and astrocytes (Kempski et al., 1988) on extracellular acidification. Interestingly, a normal volume of C6 glioma cells is maintained during complete interruption of energy metabolism induced by hypoxia (disabling the Na^+/K^+ pump) plus inhibition of glycolysis (Kempski et al., 1987). Thus, tissue acidosis and not hypoxia *per se* is a more significant factor to control to limit cell swelling.

With reference again to the brain ischemia model of Bednar and coworkers (1991), they kept systemic pH constant throughout the experiment but did not measure local pH changes in the brain which may have been highly acidic in and around the infarct region. Acidotic swelling of brain cells could increase tissue volume and force the vascular volume to decrease (total brain volume = tissue volume + vascular volume is constant), thereby compressing blood vessels and restricting flow. This effect could furthermore be compounded by the capillary EC swelling described above. Over time with a dwindling energy supply, cellular pH regulation and other vital processes will be compromised with eventual irreversible cell death.

WBC INVOLVEMENT

The WBCs have been implicated as playing a possible hemodynamic role in the no-reflow phenomenon by virtue of their stiff deformability and relatively large size. If trapped in the capillaries, they may become activated and release potentially toxic substances such as oxygen free radicals which are known to induce cellular injury. Also, activated cells can adhere to the endothelium of postcapillary venules, which may both increase resistance by reducing the vessel lumen and increase microvascular permeability (Grisham et al., 1986). Fluid leakage into the brain would cause edema, raise ICP, and reciprocally compress the blood volume space. Such a "compartment syndrome" has been classically described for skeletal muscle.

WBC depletion abolished the no-reflow phenomenon in skeletal muscle (Korthius et al., 1988) and attenuated it in the brain along with the maintenance of ICP and a reduced infarct size (Bednar et al., 1991). These results alone do not identify what effect, either hemodynamic or biochemical, the cells are imposing during reperfusion. And indirectly, anoxic reperfusion also minimized the no-reflow phenomenon, presumably by reducing the production of toxic oxygen metabolites (Korthuis et al., 1989). There is some evidence linking the oxygen free radical generation by WBCs to the pathogenesis of cellular function during reperfusion (Yokota et al., 1989).

WBC-ENDOTHELIUM INTERACTION

Cerebral ischemia/reperfusion injury resembles that of inflamed tissue which suggests that WBCs are involved in a capacity beyond mere physical presence. The process by which WBCs are recruited to sites of inflammation can be divided into three stages. First, the cells initially attach and roll on the endothelial wall after they are pushed there by the faster RBCs moving out of the capillaries. Secondly, the cells are activated and firmly adhere to the endothelium. And finally, the cells extravasate to the surrounding tissue. These processes are mediated by multiple adhesion molecules, with recent experimental evidence to suggest that the selectins are involved in rolling and the integrin receptors participate in the adhesion and extravasation. The endothelium also actively participates in adhesion through selectin and immunoglobulin receptor molecules. A comprehensive, up-to-date review of leukocyte-endothelium adhesion theory is available with information provided by researchers at the forefront of the field (Harlan and Liu, 1992).

"ANTI-ADHESION" THERAPY - MONOCLONAL ANTIBODIES

The inhibition of WBC adherence to the endothelium is a novel and relatively new approach to treating inflammatory disorders with the goal of minimizing tissue injury. In a skeletal muscle ischemia/reperfusion model, there was no apparent no-reflow damage when WBCs were prevented from adhering by a monoclonal antibody to the integrin receptor CD18 on the WBC (Carden et al., 1990). Similar findings in a number of other tissue models are described in the review cited above. In a set of studies by Vedder and colleagues, it was found that CD18 monoclonal antibody treatment dramatically reduced injury and improved survival in rabbits if given either prior to hemorrhagic shock (Vedder et al., 1988) or at the time of resuscitation (Vedder et al., 1989). This interesting result of effective treatment at the time of resuscitation with complete survival in the monoclonal treated group as opposed to the untreated group has been confirmed in a primate model (Mileski et al., 1990). In the only reported use of anti-adhesion therapy in a central nervous system/ischemia model, Clark et al. (1991) used a monoclonal antibody to the intercellular adhesion molecule (ICAM) on endothelium which is necessary for WBC binding. Treatment prior to ischemia had a protective effect on neurological function in their reversible spinal cord ischemia model, but not in the irreversible brain ischemia model. Thus, anti-adhesive therapy for ischemia/reperfusion conditions may be very beneficial in mitigating the deleterious consequences of WBC-EC interaction.

SUMMARY

The clinical objective for the treatment of ischemia has traditionally been to simply reinstate sufficient flow. More and more evidence, however, suggests that this is a shortsighted approach which may only lead to a worsening of the problem. Understanding the pathophysiology involved in ischemia has identified potential routes of intervention to prevent or arrest tissue injury. Two examples of such beneficial treatment and the theory and data to support their use have been described in this chapter. To recapitulate, it has been shown that reperfusion with hyperosmotic solutions opens up capillaries narrowed by swollen endothelial cells allowing a return of flow homogeneity and unobstructed WBC transit. The response is rapid and accomplishes systemic as well as microcirculatory hemodynamic normalization. Both characteristics of hyperosmotic resuscitation are distinct advantages over conventional isotonic fluid or blood reperfusion. Another mode of ischemia therapy having initial success is the use of monoclonal antibodies as an anti-adhesive therapy to inhibit intercellular binding between WBCs and microvascular endothelium. This transient suppression of the inflammatory process, otherwise initiated in ischemia and/or reperfusion, facilitates organ recovery of function with minimal untoward effects. Looking towards the future, a synergistic treatment may be the combination of hyperosmotic fluid and monoclonal antibody. The idea would be to rev up flow for a quick and universal delivery of monoclonals and other soluble mediators to their sites of action. The efficacy of these approaches for routine clinical therapy will be determined through further investigation in ischemia/reperfusion models of the brain and other organs.

REFERENCES

1.   Ames III, A., R. L. Wright, M. Kowada, J. M. Thurston, and G. Majno. Cerebral ischemia. II. The no-reflow phenomenon. *Am. J. Path.* 52: 437-447, 1968.

2.   Amundson, B., E. Jennische, and H. Haljam e. Correlative analysis of microcirculatory and cellular metabolic events in skeletal muscle during hemorrhagic shock. *Acta Physiol. Scand.* 108: 147-158, 1980a.

3.   Amundson, B., E. Jennische, and H. Haljam e. Skeletal muscle microcirculatory and cellular metabolic effects of whole blood, Ringer's acetate, and dextran 70 infusions in hemorrhagic shock. *Circ. Shock* 7: 111-120, 1980b.

4.   Bagge, U., B. Amundson, and C. Lauritzen. White blood cell deformability and plugging of skeletal muscle capillaries in hemorrhagic shock. *Acta Physiol. Scand.* 180: 159-163, 1980.

5.   Barroso-Aranda, J., G. W. Schmid-Schonbein, B. W. Zweifach, and R. L. Engler. Granulocytes and no-reflow phenomenon in irreversible hemorrhagic shock. *Circ. Res.* 63: 437-447, 1988.

6.   Bednar, M. M., S. Raymond, T. McAuliffe, P. A. Lodge, and C. E. Gross. The role of neutrophils and platelets in a rabbit model of thromboembolic stroke. *Stroke* 22: 44-50, 1991.

7.   Cala, P. M., S. E. Anderson, and E. J. Cragoe. Na/H exchange-dependent cell volume and pH regulation and disturbances. *Comp. Biochem. Physiol.* 90A: 551-555, 1988.

8.   Carden, D. L., J. K. Smith, and R. J. Korthuis. Neutrophil-mediated microvascular dysfunction in postischemic canine skeletal muscle. *Circ. Res.* 66: 1436-1444, 1990.

9.   Clark, W. M., K. P. Madden, R. Rothlein, and J. A. Zivin. Reduction of central nervous system ischemic injury by monoclonal antibody to intercellular adhesion molecule. *Stroke* 22: 877-883, 1991.

10.   Engler, R. L., G. W. Schmid-Schonbein, and R. S. Pavelec. Leukocyte capillary plugging in myocardial ischemia and reperfusion in the dog. *Am. J. Pathol.* 111: 98-111, 1983.

11.   Flores, J., D. R. DiBona, C. H. Beck, and A. Leaf. The role of cell swelling in ischemic renal damage and the protective effect of hypertonic solute. *J. Clin. Invest.* 51: 118-126, 1972.

12.   Frega, N. S., D. R. DiBona, B. Guertler, and A. Leaf. Ischemic renal injury. *Kidney Int.* 10: 17-25, 1976.

13.   Frelin, C., P. Vigne, P. Barbry, and M. Lazdunski. Molecular properties of amiloride action and of its Na^+ transporting targets. *Kid. Int.* 32: 785-793, 1987.

14.   Gidlof, A., F. Hammersen, J. Larsson, D. H. Lewis, and S.-O. Liljedahl. Is capillary endothelium in human skeletal muscle an ischemic tissue? In: *Induced Skeletal Muscle Ischemia in Man*, edited by D. H. Lewis. New York: Karger, 1982, p. 63-79.

15.   Gidlof, A., D. H. Lewis, and F. Hammersen. The effect of prolonged total ischemia on the ultrastructure of human skeletal muscle capillaries. A morphometric analysis. *Int. J. Microcirc.: Clin. Exp.* 7: 67-86, 1987.

16.   Grisham, M. B., L. A. Hernandez, and D. N. Granger. Xanthine oxidase and neutrophil infiltration in intestinal ischemia. *Am. J. Physiol.* 251: H456-G474, 1986.

17.   GrRgaard, B., L. Schürer, B. Gerdin, and K.-E. Arfors. Delayed hypoperfusion after incomplete forebrain ischemia in the rat. The role of polymorphonuclear leukocytes. *J. Cereb. Blood Flow Metab.* 9: 500-505, 1989.

18.   Gunnar, W., O. Jonasson, G. Merlotti, J. Stone, and J. Barrett. Head injury and hemorrhagic shock: Studies of the blood brain barrier and intracranial pressure after resuscitation with normal saline solution, 3% saline solution, and dextran-40. *Surgery* 103: 398-407, 1988.

19.   Gunnar, W. P., G. J. Merlotti, O. Jonasson, and J. Barrett. Resuscitation from hemorrhagic shock: Alterations of the intracranial pressure after normal saline, 3% saline, and dextran-40. *Ann. Surg.* 204: 686-692, 1986.

20.   Harlan, J. M., and D. Y. Liu, editors. *Adhesion: Its Role in Inflammatory Disease*. New York: W. H. Freeman and Company, 1992.

21.   Holcroft, J. W., M. J. Vassar, J. E. Turner, R. W. Derlet, and G. C. Kramer. 3% NaCl and 7.5% NaCl/dextran 70 in the resuscitation of severely injured patients. *Ann. Surg.* 206: 279-288, 1987.

22.   Jakubovicz, D. E., S. Grinstein, and A. Klip. Cell swelling following recovery from acidification in C6 glioma cells: an in vitro model of postischemic brain edema. *Brain Res.* 435: 138-146, 1987.

23.   Jakubovicz, D. E., and A. Klip. Lactic acid-induced swelling in C6 glial cells via Na^+/H^+ exchange. *Brain Res.* 485: 215-224, 1989.

24.   Kempski, O., F. Staub, M. Jansen, F. Schodel, and A. Baethmann. Glial swelling during extracellular acidosis in vitro. *Stroke* 19: 385-392, 1988.

25.   Kempski, O., M. Zimmer, A. Neu, F. v Rosen, M. Jansen, and A. Baethmann. Control of glial cell volume in anoxia: In vitro studies on ischemic cell swelling. *Stroke* 18: 623-628, 1987.

26.   Kloner, R. A., C. E. Ganote, D. A. Whalen, and R. B. Jennings. Effect of a transient period of ischemia on myocardial cells. II. Fine structure during the first few minutes of reflow. *Am. J. Physiol.* 74: 399-422, 1974.

27.   Korthuis, R. J., M. B. Grisham, and D. N. Granger. Leukocyte depletion attenuates vascular injury in postischemic skeletal muscle. *Am. J. Physiol.* 254: H823-H827, 1988.

28.   Korthuis, R. J., J. K. Smith, and D. L. Carden. Hypoxic reperfusion attenuates postischemic microvascular injury. *Am. J. Physiol.* 256: H315-H319, 1989.

29. Kreimeier, U., and K. Messmer. New perspectives in resuscitation and prevention of multiple organ system failure. In: *Surgical Research: Recent Concepts and Results*, edited by A. Baethmann and K. Messmer. Berlin: Springer-Verlag, 1987, p. 39-50.

30. Lewis, D. H. The response of the microvasculature in skeletal muscle to hemorrhage, trauma, and ischemia. In: *Skeletal Muscle Microcirculation, Prog. Appl. Microcirc.* 5, edited by F. Hammersen and K. Messmer, Basel: Karger, 1984, p. 127-138.

31. Maningas, P. A., L. R. DeGuzman, F. J. Tillman, C. S. Hinson, K. J. Priegnitz, K. A. Volk, and R. F. Bellamy. Small-volume infusion of 7.5% NaCl in 6% dextran 70 for the treatment of severe hemorrhagic shock in swine. *Ann. Emerg. Med.* 15: 1131-1137, 1986.

32. Maningas, P. A., K. L. Mattox, P. E. Pepe, R. L. Jones, D. V. Feliciano, and J. M. Burch. Hypertonic saline-dextran solutions for the pre-hospital management of traumatic hypotension. *Am. J. Surg.* 157: 528-534, 1989.

33. Mazzoni, M. C., P. Borgstrom, K.-E. Arfors, and M. Intaglietta. Dynamic fluid redistribution in hyperosmotic resuscitation of hypovolemic hemorrhage. *Am. J. Physiol.* 255: H629-H637, 1988.

34. Mazzoni, M. C., P. Borgstrom, M. Intaglietta, and K.-E. Arfors. Lumenal narrowing and endothelial cell swelling in skeletal muscle capillaries during hemorrhagic shock. *Circ. Shock* 29: 27-39, 1989.

35. Mazzoni, M. C., P. Borgstrom, M. Intaglietta, and K.-E. Arfors. Capillary narrowing in hemorrhagic shock is rectified by hyperosmotic saline-dextran reinfusion. *Circ. Shock* 31: 407-418, 1990.

36. Mazzoni, M. C., M. Intaglietta, E. J. Cragoe, and K.-E. Arfors. Amiloride-sensitive Na^+ pathways in capillary endothelial cell swelling during hemorrhagic shock. *J. Appl. Physiol.*, in press, 1992.

37. Menger, M. D., F.-U. Sack, J. H. Barker, G. Feifel, and K. Messmer. Quantitative analysis of microcirculatory disorders after prolonged ischemia in skeletal muscle: Therapeutic effects of prophylactic isovolemic hemodilution. *Res. Exp. Med.* 188: 151-165, 1988.

38. Mileski, W. J., R. K. Winn, N. B. Vedder, T. H. Pohlman, J. M. Harlan, and C. L. Rice. Inhibition of CD18-dependent neutrophil adherence reduces organ injury after hemorrhagic shock in primates. *Surgery* 108: 206-212, 1990.

39. Nakayama, S., G. C. Kramer, R. C. Carlsen, J. W. Holcroft. Infusion of very hypertonic saline to bled rats: membrane potentials and fluid shifts. *J. Surg. Res.* 38: 180-186, 1985.

40.   Prough, D. S., J. C. Johnson, G. V. Poole, E. H. Stullken, W. E. Johnstron, and R. Royster. Effects of intracranial pressure of resuscitation from hemorrhagic shock with hypertonic saline versus lactated Ringer's solution. *Crit. Care Med.* 13: 407-411, 1985.

41.   Shires, G. T., J. N. Cunningham, C. R. F. Baker, S. F. Reeder, H. Illner, I. Y. Wagner, J. Maher. Alterations in cellular membrane function during hemorrhagic shock in primates. *Ann. Surg.* 176: 288-295, 1972.

42.   Siesjo, B. K. Historical overview. Calcium, ischemia, and death of brain cells. *Ann. NY Acad. Sci.* 522: 638-661, 1988.

43.   Smith, G. J., G. C. Kramer, P. Perron, S. Nakayama, R. A. Gunther, and J. W. Holcroft. A comparison of several hypertonic solutions for resuscitation of bled sheep. *J. Surg. Res.* 39: 517-528, 1985.

44.   Vedder, N. B., B. W. Fouty, R. K. Winn, J. M. Harlan, and C. L. Rice. Role of neutrophils in generalized reperfusion injury associated with resuscitation from shock. *Surgery* 106: 509-516, 1989.

45.   Vedder, N. B., R. K. Winn, C. L. Rice, E. Y. Chi, K.-E. Arfors, and J. M. Harlan. A monoclonal antibody to the adherence-promoting leukocyte glycoprotein, CD18, reduces organ injury and improves survival from hemorrhagic shock and resuscitation in rabbits. *J. Clin. Invest.* 81: 939-944, 1988.

46.   Warnke, K. C., and T. C. Skalak. The effects of leukocytes on blood flow in a model skeletal muscle capillary network. *Microvasc. Res.* 40: 118-136, 1990.

47.   Weiloch, T. Neuronal injury and cerebrovascular disorders. *Current Opinion in Neurology and Neurosurgery* 3: 944-950, 1990.

48.   Yokota, J., J. P. Minei, G. A. Fantini, and G. T. Shires. Role of leukocytes in reperfusion injury of skeletal muscle after partial ischemia. *Am. J. Physiol.* 257: H1068-H1075, 1989.

4

EVALUATION AND TREATMENT OF THE PATIENT WITH AN ACUTE ISCHEMIC INFARCTION

Dara G. Jamieson, M.D.

Assistant Professor of Neurology
Temple University School of Medicine
Philadelphia, PA *

Approximately 500,000 new cases of stroke occur in the United States every year (6). Up to 85% of patients survive a stroke, depending on its cause, making stroke the most common cause of morbidity in the US. (45,74,118). Although the risk of having a stroke increases with increasing age it can occur in the neonate as well as the older individual. Stroke is becoming increasingly frequent in young adults; however, it remains a group of disorders usually seen in the elderly in association with other medical illnesses. The incidence of stroke may have been declining (45,74); however, as the average age of the population increases the number of people at risk for stroke will increase. The economic costs of stroke is enormous with a cost of an estimated $15 billion a year in health costs and lost productivity alone (6).

"Stroke" generally refers to the acute onset of neurological deficits due to cerebral damage caused by the disruption of blood flow within the brain. This non-specific term includes ischemic (bland) or hemorrhagic infarction due to thromboembolic disease, as well as subarachnoid hemorrhage and intracerebral (parenchymal) hemorrhage (119). The initial management and

---

* Current address: Department of Neurology, Pennsylvania Hospital, 8th and Spruce Streets, Philadelphia, PA   19107

evaluation of stroke due to ischemic infarction differs from that of subarachnoid or intracerebral hemorrhage and this review will concentrate on the causes, prevention and management of ischemic cerebral infarction.

THE ETIOLOGY OF ISCHEMIC CEREBRAL INFARCTION

The most common causes of ischemic cerebral infarction are thromboembolic atherosclerotic disease of the extracranial (i.e. the carotid arteries or the vertebrobasilar system) or intracranial vessels and occlusion of intracranial or extracranial vessels by emboli from the heart. The greatest risk factors for cerebral infarction are advanced age and a prior infarction or episode of transient ischemia. Other major risk factors include hypertension, diabetes, cigarette smoking, and cardiac disease.

ATHEROSCLEROTIC DISEASE OF CRANIAL VESSELS

Atherosclerosis preferentially involves the aorta, the coronary arteries, and both intracranial and extracranial arteries. The earliest lesion of atherosclerosis is the development of fatty streaks, made up of lipid-laden foam cells, in the arterial intimal surface (20). The fibrous plaque which develops in more circumscribed locations consists of a smooth muscle cell and collagen matrix, with macrophages and lymphocytes. There is a central region of cellular debris, lipid and cholesterol crystals. Complicated plaques may contain hemosiderin and areas of calcification. The denuded endothelial surface may serve as a focus for platelet accumulation leading to thrombus formation with embolization or vessel stenosis. Primary intraplaque hemorrhage may also lead to luminal thrombosis and embolization. The factors which initiate the production of symptomatic atherosclerotic plaque formation are unknown although advanced age, hypertension, diabetes, and elevated serum lipids may accelerate the process.

Accelerated carotid artery atherosclerosis has been noted in the radiation field after therapeutic neck irradiation (24). The time between the radiation and the development of an infarction is usually on the order of years.

Cerebral infarction in the setting of extracranial cervical vessel atherosclerosis is complex and incompletely understood. Infarction may be due to stenosis resulting in thrombus formation either at the site of stenosis or distally. The thrombus then produces intracranial or extracranial occlusion either directly or by embolization. Hemodynamic compromise can also result in cerebral infarction due to significant decrease in systemic blood pressure in the setting of hemodynamically significant extracranial vessel stenosis. The adequacy of intracranial and extracranial collateral circulation probably plays a significant role in determining the extent and location of such an infarction.

The source of vessel occlusion, thrombotic or embolic, is difficult to determine clinically although thrombotic disease of the cranial vessels may cause the stuttering onset of a neurologic deficit or a neurologic deficit present on awakening.

CARDIAC DISEASE AND STROKE

Approximately 20% of strokes are due to emboli from a cardiac source (20). Infarction due to intracranial vessel occlusion from a cardioembolic source often presents with the abrupt onset of maximal neurologic deficit. Arrhythmia such as atrial fibrillation and "sick sinus syndrome" are associated with an increased risk of cerebral infarction. Valvular disease due to rheumatic fever or subacute bacterial endocarditis and prosthetic valves are sources of emboli. The incidence of neurologic complications in infective endocarditis is between 27 and 39% and a neurologic complication may be the presenting symptom in 12-17% of patients (109). Cardiac wall hypokinesis in the setting of cardiomyopathy, a recent myocardial infarction, or congenital heart disease may be a setting for intracardiac thrombi which can embolize. Less commonly emboli from atrial myxomas or "paradoxical" emboli from a venous source through an atrial or ventricular septal defect can cause distal intracranial or extracranial arterial occlusion (42). Emboli due to Libman-Sacks endocarditis are a major cause of stroke in systemic lupus erythematosus (31, 43).

Cerebral infarction can be seen as a complication of cardiac surgery including transplantation, cardiac catheterization, transluminal angioplasty, or pump oxygenation. The reported incidence of neurologic complications of open-heart surgery varies widely, ranging from 7 to 61% for transient and from 1.6 to 23% for permanent complications (51). The 2 to 5% incidence of cerebral infarction seen after cardiac surgery is felt to be related in most cases to microemboli rather than a low flow state secondary to carotid stenosis (44). Microvascular abnormalities have been show to correlate with cardiopulmonary bypass (91). Sources of emboli include embolization from atherosclerosis or thrombus at the arterial cannulation site, air, fat, talc, left ventricular thrombus, or aortic dissection. A prior history of cerebral infarction is the most significant risk for intraoperative complications.

OTHER RISK FACTORS FOR STROKE

Cigarette smoking has been demonstrated to be an independent risk factor for stroke (82). In the Honolulu Heart Program cigarette smoking men had a two to three times increased risk of thromboembolic or hemorrhagic stroke, independent of other risk factors, than did nonsmokers (1). Cessation of smoking significantly decreased this risk over the 12 year follow-up period. The Nurses' Health Study also showed an increased risk of stroke in female nurses who smoked, with increased number of cigarettes being associated with increased risk (22). The Framingham Study found that the stroke risk in smokers who quit reached the level of nonsmokers by five years after cessation (130).

The correlation between alcohol consumption and stroke risk remains controversial. Epidemiological evidence indicates that excessive alcohol consumption is a risk factor for both ischemic and hemorrhagic cerebrovascular disease (54). The association between moderate consumption and ischemic cerebral infarction is less clear, although there may be the protective effect proposed for coronary artery disease (19).

Cerebral infarction is seen in association with intravenous drug use, due to primary effects of the drug itself, the dilutant, or as a result of valvular disease (17). Association has been noted between cerebral infarction and cocaine use (29, 76, 80). Cerebral infarction is one of many neurologic complications of acquired immunodeficiency syndrome (35).

Acute severe hypotension, such as during cardiac arrest, can result in cerebral infarction. When hypotension occurs with severe atherosclerotic disease of extracranial vessels a "watershed" infarction in overlapping vascular territories (e.g. middle cerebral and anterior cerebral arteries) may result.

Dissection of extracranial vessels is a not uncommon cause of cerebral infarction in all age groups (90). Although most cases are probably spontaneous, some cases of vertebral artery dissection occur after neck manipulation (47). There may be association with underlying arterial abnormalities such as fibromuscular dysplasia or pseudoxanthoma elasticum or vascular anomalies.

Central nervous system (CNS) vasculitis, with inflammation and necrosis of blood vessels and tissue ischemia, can be isolated angiitis with vascular changes confined to the CNS; part of multiple, systemic vasculitides; or secondary to a variety of systemic disorders (61). Isolated angiitis of the CNS can present with neurologic symptoms which can be acute or subacute; focal, multifocal, or diffuse. Granulomata or giant cells are a common, but not absolute, finding on histopathologic examination. Systemic necrotizing arteridites, which can involve the CNS, include polyarteritis nodosa, Wegner's granulomatosis, sarcoidosis, and lymphomatoid granulomatosis. Autoimmune and infectious diseases, neoplasms, and toxins can secondarily cause CNS vasculitis.

Venous infarction can result from inflammatory lesions of veins, which can be of infectious origin. Noninfectious causes of venous infarction include dehydration; hypercoagulable states, including those associated with pregnancy or neoplasms; and drugs.

Hematologic disorders and coagulopathies predisposing to thrombosis may account for approximately 4% of infarctions in young adults (57). Inherited deficiencies of coagulation inhibitors such as antithrombin III, protein C, protein S, and heparin cofactor II have been associated clinically with thrombosis. Inherited abnormalities of fibrinolysis have also been linked to thrombosis. Antiphospholipid antibodies have been associated with a tendency toward venous and arterial thrombosis. A subset of these acquired immunoglobulins, lupus anticoagulants, result in a prolonged activated partial thromboplastin time (aPTT) and have been associated with cerebral infarction as well as other neurologic abnormalities (13). Anticardiolipin antibodies have been assayed by various methods with prevalence in two studies of 29% (77) and 8.2% (IgG), 9.1% (IgM) (66) in patients with cerebral ischemia. Polycythemia, either due to a primary myeloproliferative stem cell disorder, or secondary to congenital heart disease, dehydration or smoking may increase the risk of thrombosis (62). Cerebral ischemia may occur in approximately 15% of patients with sickle cell anemia. Ischemic infarction is more common in children with sickle cell disease whereas, cerebral hemorrhage is more common in young adults. Cerebral infarction may be more common in individuals with sickle cell trait and beta-thalassemia. Thrombocytopenia, disseminated intravascular coagulation, and thrombotic thrombocytopenic purpura (TTP) also predispose to cerebral infarction. TTP may be one of the major causes of cerebral infarction in patients with systemic lupus erythematosus.

Genetic predisposition to stroke occurs (5,96). Hereditary cardiac conduction diseases, cardiomyopathies and other familial cardiac conditions may predispose to embolic infarction. Thromboembolic infarctions are associated with homocystinuria, Fabry's disease, and neurocutaneous syndromes. Many of the hemoglobinopathies, platelet defects, and coagulopathies which predispose to infarction are hereditary. Mitochondrial disorders which appear to follow a maternal inheritance pattern are associated with cerebral infarction. Abnormalities of vessel wall predisposing to cerebral infarction can occur in Marfan's syndrome, pseudoxanthoma elasticum, and Ehlers-Danlos syndrome.

CEREBRAL INFARCTION IN YOUNG PEOPLE

The etiologies of cerebral infarction in a young patient (< 50 years of age) may be more varied than in older individuals (9,12,75). Atherosclerosis, a major cause of cerebral infarction in the elderly, is less often a factor in young patients. Cardiac causes such as congenital heart disease, mitral valve prolapse, and endocarditis, both infectious and non-infectious, should be considered in every young patient. Arterial dissection, with or without antecedent trauma, may be a cause of infarction in these patients. Coagulation disturbances are recognized as a major cause of either arterial or venous cerebral infarction. Antiphospholipid syndrome should be considered in a young patient with an unexplained cerebral infarction (13). The correlation between migraine and cerebral infarction has been noted (97), although other factors such as hypertension, smoking and oral contraception use may also be significant (23).

Pregnancy and the postpartum period may be associated with an increased risk for either intracranial venous or arterial occlusion (127). Estrogens may produce changes in blood coagulability and platelet functioning and may have direct effects on blood vessels. Aseptic intracranial venous thrombosis may occur anytime in pregnancy although it is usually seen in the third trimester or postpartum period or in association with preeclampsia. The usual causes for cerebral infarction in a young person may also be seen in pregnant women. Other causes unique to pregnancy include emboli due to amniotic fluid, air or fat.

EVALUATION OF A PATIENT WITH AN ACUTE CEREBRAL INFARCTION

GENERAL HISTORY AND EXAMINATION

An extensive history of the presenting complaint as well as the past medical history and family history must be elicited from every patient or the patient's family. The general examination of a patient with a cerebral infarction should include evaluation for asymmetries of brachial artery pressures and for orthostatic blood pressure and pulse changes. Asymmetry of the brachial or radial pulses should be assessed. Carotid arteries should be palpated and auscultated in the neck. Auscultation of the heart for murmurs, clicks or arrhythmias is essential. The skin should be examined for evidence of cyanosis, rashes or hemorrhage. Evidence of recent or prior, head or neck trauma or surgery should be noted.

NEUROLOGIC EXAMINATION

The cause of a cerebral infarction can often be inferred from the general medical and neurologic history. The time course of the neurologic abnormality must be precisely defined as different time periods and patterns of ischemia have different prognostic and therapeutic implications. A pattern of recent, frequent episodes of transient neurologic deficit represents a greater risk for imminent cerebral infarction than does an isolated episode in the past. By convention a transient ischemic attack (TIA) is defined as a neurologic deficit of abrupt onset and brief duration lasting less than 24 hours. Most TIAs last 2 to 15 minutes. The longer the duration of the TIA the greater the likelihood of finding an appropriate area of infarction on CT or MRI. Approximately 20% of thromboembolic infarctions are preceded by TIAs (6). Different therapy may be indicated for a cerebral infarction with worsening deficit than for an infarction with maximal deficit at onset.

A complete, thorough and meticulously documented neurologic examination is absolutely essential to diagnose cerebrovascular disease and to monitor response to treatment. Assessing the level of consciousness is an essential part of the neurologic examination as progressive lethargy may indicate the development of life threatening cerebral edema. A mental status examination directed toward language and spatial abnormalities can indicate which hemisphere is damaged. A thorough fundoscopic examination should be done to look for platelet-fibrin or cholesterol emboli in the retina as well as to examine the optic disk for signs of increased intracranial pressure.

Some signs such as hemiparesis, hemisensory loss, dysarthria, or hemianopic defect can be due to either carotid artery or vertebrobasilar territory disease but other signs can indicate which vascular territory is involved. Monocular visual loss, aphasia, and cognitive or behavioral abnormalities may indicate carotid artery territory disease whereas, nausea, vomiting, vertigo, limb or gait ataxia, double vision due to eye movement abnormalities, palatal dysfunction, and simultaneous bilateral or crossed motor and sensory abnormalities may indicate vertebrobasilar territory disease.

DIFFERENTIAL DIAGNOSIS

Other causes of acute onset of neurologic abnormalities must be differentiated from cerebral infarctions. Hemorrhage into brain parenchyma presents with signs and symptoms which are generally indistinguishable from those seen in infarction (38). Intracranial hemorrhage may be accompanied by a headache or impaired level of consciousness. Extremely high blood pressure is often seen at the onset of symptoms. The most common causes of intraparenchymal hemorrhage are hypertension; vasculitis; arteriovenous malformations; trauma; coagulation abnormalities, either primary or drug induced; and aneurysms. The locations of hypertensive hemorrhages are generally subcortical (e.g. putamenal, thalamic, white matter), brainstem (e.g. pontine), or cerebellar. Intracerebral or dural tumors, both primary and metastatic, can hemorrhage. Lobar hemorrhage due to amyloid angiopathy may be seen in association with dementia in the elderly.

Extraparenchymal hemorrhage may be due to trauma or vascular abnormalities. The degree of trauma associated with subdural or epidural hematomas may be mild or massive. Subdural hematomas are due to tearing of the bridging veins or pial arteries resulting in the collection of blood between the dura and the pia. They may be acute with symptoms presenting within hours to days or chronic with the presentation of symptoms weeks to years after the inciting trauma. The treatment of acute subdural hematomas is generally surgical evacuation whereas treatment of a chronic subdural must be individualized.

When subarachnoid hemorrhage (SAH) presents with focal neurologic abnormalities it may appear to be an ischemic infarction. SAH is usually associated, however, with the acute onset of a severe headache and stiff neck with or without altered level of consciousness. The symptoms at the onset of a SAH are generally severe; however, occasionally they are so mild as to make the diagnosis elusive (3). Seizures may occur during the acute phase of SAH. Infarction due to vasospasm is a common complication seen after the first few days after a subarachnoid bleed. The risk of infarction increases with increased amount of subarachnoid blood and may represent vascular response to injury caused by vasoreactive substances. Saccular aneurysms, trauma, and arteriovenous malformations are the most common causes of SAH.

Seizures, particularly when there is a prolonged postictal abnormality without obvious tonic-clonic motor manifestations, may appear similar to transient ischemia. Metabolic encephalopathy, focal encephalitis and tumor must be considered in the differential diagnosis of transient neurologic abnormalities. Rarely, conversion reaction or malingering may be confused with a cerebral infarction.

LABORATORY AND RADIOLOGIC EVALUATION

All patients suspected of having had a cerebral infarction should have routine blood work including glucose, electrolytes, renal and liver function tests, complete blood count with white cell differential and platelets. Serum cholesterol and triglyceride levels, with fractionation of cholesterol if it is elevated, should be ordered. Prothrombin time and activated partial thromboplastin time should be assessed. If they are abnormal or there is a suspicion of a hypercoaguable state other tests such as anticardiolipin antibody, lupus inhibitor (Kaolin clotting time, dilute Russell viper venom time), protein S, protein C and antithrombin III levels should be obtained. A sedimentation rate and RPR are used to screen for syphilis, vasculitis, infection or collagen vascular disease. A urine and blood screen for drugs, both therapeutic and illicit, and HIV antibody titers may be indicated.

An electrocardiogram (ECG) is essential for all patients. In many elderly patients serial ECGs and cardiac enzymes should be ordered to rule out a concomitant myocardial infarction. Because coronary artery atherosclerosis is found very frequently in patients with atherosclerotic cerebrovascular disease it may be appropriate to evaluate some patients by nuclear cardiology perfusion imaging for significant coronary artery disease (123, 33). Evaluation for asymptomatic coronary artery disease may also be warranted because of the strong association with carotid artery disease (21).

An uncontrasted CT scan of the brain is essential to rule out other causes of acute onset neurologic abnormality such as hemorrhage. Parenchymal hemorrhage and blood in the subarachnoid space, cisterns, or ventricles must be examined for carefully. The CT scan in ischemic cerebral infarction may be normal within the first 12-24 hours after the onset of symptoms and a repeat scan in a few days may be necessary (59).

Carotid duplex Doppler, combining carotid realtime ultrasound sonography and Doppler spectral analysis, is a convenient, noninvasive method to screen for carotid artery stenosis, carotid artery dissection or fibromuscular dysplasia in the region of the common carotid artery, bifurcation, and proximal internal and external carotid arteries (39,55). Oculoplethesmography can indicate asymmetry of ophthalmic artery pressures as seen in hemodynamically significant internal carotid artery stenosis. Transcranial Doppler (TCD) is a noninvasive ultrasound technique using pulsed wave Doppler to screen for patients with intracranial and extracranial arterial disease and to monitor changes over time (32,99,126). It can be used to localize areas of focal stenosis within major intracranial vessels, such as the internal carotid artery siphon; the middle, anterior and posterior cerebral arteries; the basilar artery; and the intracranial vertebral arteries. TCD is very useful for assessing collateralization due to hemodynamically significant internal carotid artery stenosis and can often confirm a suspicious area seen on carotid duplex Doppler. Reversal of flow direction within the ophthalmic artery, seen by placing the ultrasound probe above the closed eye, may indicate external carotid artery collateralization due to a hemodynamically significant lesion of the ipsilateral internal carotid artery. Increased flow velocity in the contralateral anterior cerebral artery can indicate collateralization through the anterior communicating artery from the intact to the compromised hemisphere. TCD can document, at bedside, vasospasm of major intracranial vessels in SAH. Advances in TCD now permit two-dimensional color-coded real time images of intravascular flow in the basal cerebral arteries (111a). Characteristic wave formations can be seen using TCD in brain death (93).

Other studies are done as warranted. Magnetic resonance imaging (MRI) is useful for localizing brain stem infarction, which is poorly seen on CT scan, well as for imaging diffuse periventricular white matter changes seen in chronic ischemia (73,102). MRI has superior image resolution with the ability to show smaller areas of tissue damage than does the CT scan. MRI studies of cerebral infarction done within the first few hours of the onset of symptoms show the ischemic regions as high signal intensity on T2 weighted images. Later the infarct is seen as a hyperintense signal on T2 weighted images and a hypointense signal on T1 images. When an acute intraparenchymal hemorrhage is imaged deoxyhemoglobin appears as a hypointense region on T2 weighted images (8). Subacutely, as methemoglobin forms, hyperintense signals are seen on T1 then T2 weighted images. The changes in hemoglobin composition and surrounding edema can be used to estimate the age of the hemorrhage. MRI can be used to detect blood in the cerebrospinal fluid in acute subarachnoid hemorrhage and in some cases may be superior to CT scanning in detecting aneurysms (71).

When there is concern over a cardiac source of emboli transthoracic echocardiography is essential (123). It is indicated in most young patients or when multiple or bilateral infarctions are seen in both anterior (internal carotid artery) and posterior (vertebrobasilar system) circulations. It must be done if there is a history of a myocardial infarction and in all cases of suspected cardiac or valvular disease. In cases where a cardiac source of cerebral embolus is strongly suspected, transesophageal echocardiography (TEE) may be indicated (78). In a study comparing transthoracic and transesophageal echocardiography in 63 patients with potential cardiac sources of cerebral emboli cases of atrial septal aneurysm, patent foramen ovale, left atrial appendage thrombus, and myxomatous mitral valve were found only on TEE. (28)

A twenty-four Holter monitor may be necessary if there is concern about an intermittent arrhythmia. Multiple sets of blood cultures should be drawn on all young patients with infarctions especially when multiple vascular territories are involved. Fever, malaise and heart murmur are also indications for blood cultures. Hemoglobin electrophoresis can rule out sickle cell disease as a cause of stroke. Electroencephalography is rarely indicated except in cases of suspected encephalitis. A lumbar puncture is not indicated in the evaluation of an presumed ischemic infarction unless there is concern about subarachnoid hemorrhage or meningitis. In these cases a lumbar puncture should be done emergently by someone proficient in the technique. If pheochromocytoma is of concern a 24 hour urine screen for total metanephrines or vanillymandelic acid concentrations should be obtained.

Arteriography is important in the evaluation of a patient with cerebral infarction especially when the technique is available without excessive risk to the patient. Major complications (i.e. stroke, death) occur in 1-2%, and minor complications (ie. reversible neurologic deficit, hematoma) occur in 5-6% of patients. Carotid arteriography can confirm carotid stenosis or occlusion as seen on screening carotid duplex Doppler. It can provide definitive diagnosis of extracranial or intracranial arterial dissection, vasculitis, fibromuscular dysplasia, intracranial or extracranial atherosclerotic vascular disease, arteriovenous malformations and aneurysms.

Other new neuroradiologic techniques may prove useful in the evaluation of cerebral infarction however, their availability is limited at this time. Positron emission tomography (PET) (70) has been used to document the sequential changes in local cerebral glucose metabolism (lCMRgl), blood flow oxygen metabolism (lCMRO2), and oxygen extraction seen in cerebral infarction (100,129). The best predictor of clinical outcome appears to be lCMRO2 (79) with decreases seen within 24 to 48 hours after the ictus (2). Using PET nimodipine was found to increase lCMRgl in noninfarcted brain regions in patients with cerebral infarction (64).

Magnetic resonance angiography (MRA) is a noninvasive technique which can provide both two and three dimensional images of both extracranial and intracranial cerebral circulation. Imaging of carotid bifurcation stenosis in a recent study showed sensitivity of 86% and specificity of 92% of MRA as compared to invasive angiography (72). In the evaluation of intracranial vasculature MRA may be able to detect aneurysms as small as 3-4 mm although the sensitivity varies with the technique used (107). Nuclear magnetic resonance spectroscopy (128) using phosphorus-31 can monitor intracellular pH and energy metabolites including ATP, phosphocreatine, and inorganic phosphate. 1H-NMR can provide images and monitor levels of lactate, glutamine, glutamate, and other compounds of interest in ischemia.

Single photon emission computerized tomography (SPECT) (67,85,37) is a nuclear medicine technique which can provide information on areas of decreased perfusion in the brain and may be helpful in cases of suspected transient ischemia associated with normal CT or MRI scans. The technique may have predictive value with poor clinical outcome at one month correlating with severe hypoperfusion in the affected hemisphere at six hours or less after the onset of symptoms (53). The cerebral blood flow at one week post-ictus has not been found to correlate with outcome. In a SPECT study using technetium-99m HM-PAO in patients with an episode of transient ischemia lasting less than 1 hour and greater than 75% internal carotid artery stenosis, a hypoperfusion deficit was seen in 4 of 12 patients. Three of these patients but none of the other patients subsequently developed an ipsilateral infarct 3 - 7 days later. Some episodes of transient ischemia may be associated with focal hypoperfusion which predisposes to early infarction (11).

REDUCTION OF STROKE RISK

MODIFICATION OF BEHAVIOR
Reduction of risk of cerebral infarction must begin with behavior modification. Habits known to be deleterious to cerebral vasculature such as cigarette smoking, illicit drug use, alcohol abuse, and dietary excesses should be curtailed or eliminated. Weight should be reduced as appropriate. Hypertension must be aggressively but appropriately managed. Although the correlation between elevated serum cholesterol and risk of cerebral infarction awaits elucidation there may be a role for cholesterol lowering medications in certain patients.

ANTIPLATELET MEDICATION

Aspirin
The use of platelet antiaggregant agents has focused on their role in the prevention of cerebral infarction, either primary or recurrent, rather than their use in the acute setting (47,122). Initial treatment for transient ischemic attacks is generally aspirin. The optimum dose is controversial as *in* vitro studies have shown platelet inhibition with low doses but clinical studies which have shown benefit with aspirin have used doses up to 1300 mg daily (33a).

Ticlopidine
Ticlopidine, a platelet antiaggregatory agent, may be used in patients who continue to have symptoms of ischemia on aspirin. The Ticlopidine Aspirin Stroke Study (TASS) (58,87) compared the effects of ticlopidine (500 mg daily) and aspirin (1300 mg daily) on patients who had recent transient or mildly persistent focal cerebral or retinal ischemia. There was a 12% risk reduction with ticlopidine in the three-year event rate for nonfatal stroke or death and a 21% risk reduction with ticlopidine in the three-year event rate for fatal and nonfatal strokes. The Canadian American Ticlopidine Study (CATS) (48,50) assessed the effect of ticlopidine (500 mg daily) versus placebo in the reduction of subsequent occurrence of stroke, myocardial infarction, or vascular death in patients who had had a recent thromboembolic infarct. There was a relative overall risk reduction in the event rate of 30.2% with ticlopidine. Ticlopidine carries a risk of severe but reversible neutropenia (<1%), diarrhea (20%), rash (14%)(50,58).

ANTICOAGULATION

Transient Ischemia

There may be a role for short term outpatient anticoagulation with warfarin sodium of patients with a history of "crescendo" transient ischemic attacks. This may be initiated after a course of in-hospital intravenous heparin anticoagulation. It some cases warfarin therapy can be initiated as an outpatient. Both medical and social factors must be taken into consideration before committing a patient to outpatient anticoagulation. Sources of potential complications such as gait difficulty, dementia, alcohol use, past history of poor medical compliance, and drug interactions must be assessed.

Anticoagulation and Atrial Fibrillation

The use of long-term anticoagulation in order to prevent recurrent cerebral infarction in patients with potential cardiac source of emboli has been controversial. Recent studies, however, indicate that in most cases either aspirin or warfarin should be used for infarct prophylaxis (10,98). An ongoing study in the United States of the use of aspirin or warfarin in patients with atrial fibrillation, unrelated to valvular disease, has shown decreased risk of cerebral infarction with antithrombotic therapy (121). Further analysis is ongoing in this study to determine whether aspirin or warfarin is preferable (121a, 121b). An earlier Danish study (98) compared anticoagulation with warfarin in an open trial, and aspirin and placebo in a double-blind fashion in patients with chronic non-valvular atrial fibrillation. The incidence of thromboembolic complications and vascular death were significantly lower in the warfarin group than in the aspirin and placebo groups, which did not differ significantly. Bleeding side effects were greater in the warfarin group.

Surgical Prevention of Cerebral Infarction

The role for surgery in the prevention of cerebral infarction is being actively investigated. Carotid endarterectomies have been performed for 35 years in an effort to decrease the risk of cerebral infarction by removing from the carotid arteries the presumed source of emboli, thrombus or both (104). The surgery itself, however, carries a risk of cerebral infarction; although, in selected patients at experienced centers even elderly patients can undergo the surgery with low risk (88).

The North American Symptomatic Carotid Endarterectomy Trial (NASCET) (95) is an international, multi-center trial comparing medical therapy alone to medical therapy plus carotid endarterectomy in patients who have an internal or common carotid artery lesion (30-99% luminal stenosis) which has resulted in either TIAs or a mild infarction. Patients are being followed in NASCET for five years and the outcomes of the two groups will be compared. Prior to the end of the five year period the study was terminated for those patients with high-grade stenosis (luminal diameter of 70-99%) because data indicated the clear benefit of surgery (94). Total stroke morbidity and mortality in the perioperative period was 5% in the surgical group and 3% during a comparable period in the medical group. Including early morbidity and mortality over 24% of medical patients, but only 7% of surgical patients, had experienced fatal or non-fatal ipsilateral stroke at 18 months, yielding a risk reduction of 17% (p<0.001). Among symptomatic patients with high grade stenosis carotid endarterectomy reduced the risk of major or fatal stroke in any territory or death from any cause with an absolute risk reduction of over 7% (p<0.01). Results are not yet available concerning symptomatic patients with moderate (30-70%) carotid artery stenosis.

Other trials assessing the value of carotid endarterectomy on symptomatic lesions have found similar results. The European Carotid Endarterectomy Trial showed no benefit with surgery on 0-29% stenosis; however, infarct reduction was seen when the degree of stenosis was over 69%. Data accumulation continues in the 30-69% group (36).

Trials are ongoing to asses the efficacy of carotid endarterectomy in patients who have no symptoms referable to carotid stenosis but may be at increased risk of infarction because of the presence of a significant carotid artery lesion (7). One recently conpleted trial (66a) found no surgical benefit in patients with asymptomatic disease when stroke and death alone were assessed; although, there was a decrease in outcome events when TIAs were included.

In patients with carotid artery occlusion or significant intracranial disease, anastomosis of the superficial temporal artery to the middle cerebral artery was proposed as a method to decrease risk of infarction. A randomized, multicenter trial involving 1337 patients failed to show any benefit conferred by the procedure, which is now rarely performed (34).

MANAGEMENT OF THE PATIENT WITH AN ACUTE ISCHEMIC INFARCTION

ACUTE SUPPORTIVE THERAPY

Blood Pressure Management

Acute hypertension is seen in 40-50% of patients within the first 24-48 hours after an infarction (125). The etiology of systemic blood pressure elevation is unclear with the most likely causes being a response to elevation of plasma cathecholamines (89,92) and to redistribution of cerebral blood flow in the region surrounding the infarct (113). In a study in which the strongest predictors of elevated blood pressure in stroke were prior hypertension and intracranial hemorrhage, the mental stress of hospitalization was suggested as a cause of peri-infarct hypertension (18).

In the normal brain cerebral blood flow is maintained relatively constant within a wide range of mean arterial blood pressures. In patients who are chronically hypertensive the mean arterial blood pressures between which blood flow is maintained constant are shifted to higher values. With cerebral ischemia and infarction this cerebral autoregulation is lost resulting in a more passive direct relationship between mean arterial blood pressure and cerebral blood flow. Acute reduction of blood pressure may decrease perfusion to the tissue surrounding the core of the infarct. Tissue within this "penumbra" may have reversible damage and may be able to recover metabolically if flow is not further compromised. For these reasons the elevated blood pressure, seen within the first hours to days after an infarction, may be necessary to maintain cerebral perfusion and prevent increased ischemia. It is generally agreed that great restraint must be shown in treating hypertension in the setting of an acute infarction (25,116). Agents that are rapidly reversible, such as intravenous sodium nitroprusside, and which have relatively little central effect, such as intravenous labetalol, should be used.

Because of concern about continued bleeding blood pressure management should be more aggressive in patients with intracerebral hemorrhage than with ischemic cerebral infarction, although generally only a moderate reduction in blood pressure is warranted. In subarachnoid hemorrhage hypervolemia hemodilution and drug-induced hypertension may be used to decrease the risk of vasospasm, however, the patient must be closely monitored for signs of congestive heart failure.

General Supportive Measures

Bed rest for the first few days after an infarction is dictated by blood pressure level, need for intravenous anticoagulation, and level of neurologic deficit. Measures to prevent deep vein thrombosis such as subcutaneous heparin, antiembolism stockings and relatively early mobilization should be instituted. Because of urinary dysfunction an indwelling catheter or preferably intermittent catheterization may be need.

Anticonvulsant therapy should only be given in the setting of an acute cerebral infarction if the patient experiences seizures. Patients who have had a subarachnoid hemorrhage should be placed on prophylactic anticonvulsant therapy to prevent rebleeding in the event of a seizure.

Nutrition and Fluid Balance

Close attention should be directed toward fluid and electrolyte balance since excess hydration may increase cerebral edema. Even relatively mild hyperglycemia at the time of presentation has been shown to be correlated with poor outcome (83,101). In a study in which fasting glucose and glysolated hemoglobin were assayed in patients with cerebral infarction within 48 hours of the ictus increased mortality at three months was associated with stress hyperglycemia in non-diabetics but not with elevated glucose in diabetics (132). These results may indicate that the outcome may be related to stroke severity rather than a deleterious effect of glucose on the brain. However fluid losses should be replenished with isotonic saline. In cases of severe stroke, the patient should not be fed until swallowing function can be assessed. Tube feedings may be necessary until swallowing function is regained.

Temperature Regulation
Since hyperthermia is felt to increase damage from cerebral ischemia even mild elevation in body temperature should be treated with antipyretic medication while the cause of the fever is being investigated. Because of increased age, concomitant medical illnesses, and incapacitation from the infarction these patients are at risk for pneumonia, urinary tract infections, venous thromboses, and pulmonary emboli, all of which can cause fever. "Central fever" due to hypothalamic dysfunction is often mentioned but rarely seen.

Increased Intracranial Pressure
Almost immediately after the onset of ischemia there is an increase in the water content of neurons and astrocytes due to possible dysfunction of ion exchange mechanisms. This cytotoxic edema may contribute to the initial neurologic deficit. Vasogenic edema with breakdown of cell membranes and the blood brain barrier reaches a maximum in 48-72 hours after the infarction. Steroids, however have not been found to be of benefit in the management of cerebral infarction.

In cases of massive infarction cerebral edema can result in increased intracranial pressure with herniation of brain contents through the tentorium, the faramen magnum, or across the falx. The patient may show increased lethargy, worsening of neurologic deficits, new pupillary abnormalities or changes in respiratory pattern depending on the area of the brain being compressed. This impending castrophe represents a neurologic emergency and the patient should be intubated and hyperventilated to decrease pCO2 with its vasodilatory effect. Decadron and mannitol boluses followed by maintenance doses should be given. Other methods of decreasing intracranial pressure such as fluid restriction, elevation of the head of the bed and monitoring intracranial pressure through a ventriculostomy may be needed. Blockage of cerebrospinal fluid circulation may precipitate acute hydrocephalus. In some cases, especially with large cerebellar infarcts, surgical decompression of the infarcted tissue may be necessary.

Anticoagulation
The use of heparin anticoagulation in acute cerebral infarction remains controversial (60,111). The risk of converting a nonhemorrhagic infarction to a hemorrhagic infarction is considerable and therefore anticoagulation is generally not used for completed acute ischemic infarctions. Treatment of "progressing" or "stuttering" infarction, due presumably to evolving thrombosis of major intracranial or extracranial vessels, is more problematic and there may be a role for anticoagulation in such a situation. When a completed infarction is due to an embolus from a cardiac source either in the setting of atrial fibrillation (26), valvular disease, or a left ventricular thrombus, heparin anticoagulation may play a role in preventing another

cerebral infarction in the early period of increased risk (133,134). In this situation discretion is advisable in anticoagulating massive infarctions and a period of days to a week prior to starting the anticoagulation may be warranted to minimize the risk of hemorrhagic conversion. Prior to anticoagulation sources of potential hemorrhage need to be assessed and blood pressure should be controlled. The patient must have no history of central nervous system bleeding, no active source of gastrointestinal bleeding, and adequate hepatic and renal function. The risk of inducing serious cerebral or systemic hemorrhage is 0.6% and 3% respectively (81).

Heparinoids are being evaluated as possible agents with an anticoagulant effect but a lower risk of hemorrhage.

Thrombolytic Therapy

Recently interest has been renewed in the use of thrombolytic therapy in acute cerebral infarction (15,30,117). Early studies showed serious complications with the use of exogenous agents, such as streptokinase and urokinase, by intravenous infusion. Fibrin selective agents, such as tissue plasminogen activator, are being investigated in multicenter trials to determine their usefulness in lysing clots in acute infarction (135, 136). One major difficulty with thrombolytic therapy in acute infarction is the need to institute treatment immediately after the onset of symptoms, once the CT scan has ruled out hemorrhage. Hemorrhage, both intracerebral and systemic, remains a potential complication of this treatment.

Recombinant tissue plasminogen activator (rt-PA) has a high affinity for fibrinogen and fibrin bound to plasminogen with plasmin formed in situ, reducing systemic fibrinolysis. An open multicenter angiography based study of rt-PA in patients with acute thrombotic / thromboembolic cerebral infarction is being conducted. No dose relationship of recanalization was established. Parenchymal hemorrhage, but not transformation to hemorrhagic infarction, was associated with clinical deterioration. Hemorrhagic complications were correlated with initiation of treatment at least 6 hours after the ictus (103). Further studies are ongoing.

Ancrod, which inhibits formation of cross linked fibrin and stimulates release of plasminogen activator, may result in local clot thrombolysis and is being studied in acute ischemic cerebral infarction.

The metabolic consequences of early reperfusion and the risk of hemorrhagic transformation need to be evaluated; however, thrombolytic therapy appears to be a potentially useful treatment of acute cerebral infarction.

Metabolic Therapy

Cerebral ischemia and infarction initiate a cascade of metabolic reactions resulting in cellular membrane disruption and destruction of cellular organelles (63). Much of the cellular damage appears to be mediated by calcium (113). Elevated intracellular calcium may activate lipases and proteases resulting in irreversible damage to mitochondria. Cellular membrane damage is precipitated in part by free radical production and by the effects of the activated enzymes. For these reasons there has been much recent interest in the use of calcium channel blockers in the treatment of acute cerebral ischemia (131).

Nimodipine is a calcium antagonist which acts as a cerebral vasodilator and may also have a direct neuronal effect. It has been shown to improve neurologic outcome after subarachnoid hemorrhage (105) and some studies in animal models of cerebral ischemia and infarction have indicated a beneficial effect. Gelmers et al (46) reported the results of a multicenter, double-blind, randomized, placebo-controlled study of oral nimodipine begun within 24 hours of the onset of symptoms of cerebral ischemia and given for 28 days. A significant decrease (p<0.003) in the mortality rate in men treated with nimodipine was seen. Patients with moderate-to-severe deficit at baseline showed significant improvement (p=0.003) on nimodipine. A trial (84) of 28 days of oral nimodipine versus placebo in 123 patients with an acute ischemic cerebral infarction showed no difference in overall mortality or neurologic outcome after the treatment period. When patients with moderate-to-very severe deficit were analyzed separately a statistically significant decrease in neurologic deficit (p<0.025) and a trend toward decreased mortality (12.5% in the nimodipine group; 20.8% in the placebo group) was seen in the nimodipine treated group. A large multicenter trial (124) in the United Kingdom of 120 mg daily of oral nimodipine started within 48 hours in acute cerebral infarction showed no benefit at 3 weeks or 6 months after the infarction. A large multicenter trial in the United States (14) has been conducted to further examine the effect of nimodipine in cerebral ischemia. Preliminary results indicate that the beneficial effect of nimodipine may be related to prompt treatment within 12 hours. Another multicenter trial did not show significant effect of 120 mg of oral nimodipine for acute stroke after 6 months follow-up (124). Two randomized double blind trials of intravenous nimodipine at 1 mg/hr, or 2 mg/hr or placebo for 5 days followed by oral nimodipine showed, on interim analysis, significantly worse end-of-therapy outcome in the 2 mg/hr group as compared to the placebo or 1 mg/hr groups. In patients treated within 12 hours there may have been benefit from 1mg/hr nimodipine. The Nimodipine German Austrian Stroke Trial (68) was a randomized double-blind, placebo-controlled, multi-center study of nimodipine in acute ischemic infarction. Significantly improved outcome was seen only in a subgroup of more severely affected patients on nimodipine. Further data analysis and more trials are underway. Nicardipine is an other calcium antagonist which has been shown to have possible benefit when started within 6 hours of symptoms. Hypotension must be avoided in patients treated with calcium antagonists.

The role of excitatory amino acids such as glutamate, gamma-aminobutyric acid, and N-methyl-D-aspartate (NMDA) in cerebral ischemia is being actively investigated (86). Excitatory amino acid gated channels, especially the subtype NMDA channels, appear to have a major role in mediating calcium-related neuronal damage in ischemia (27,108,110,115). NMDA channels also play a role in cellular chloride and cation influx resulting in water entry and cell lysis. Calcium entry into the cell amplifies the level of NMDA receptor activation, leading to further ion fluxes and continued cell destruction. Because of the regulating role of NMDA receptors in cell destruction in ischemia interest has focused on the use of non-competitive NMDA antagonists in cerebral infarction (115). Investigation with animal models of cerebral ischemia has shown some encouraging results although NMDA antagonists have not been shown to be of benefit in all models and may afford protection only to selected areas of the brain. Based on these results several specific NMDA antagonists; such as MK-801, dextromethorphan, dextrorphan, and ketamine; appear to show promise as therapeutic agents for clinical investigation (4,16).

Other methods of metabolic protection such as free radical scavengers have shown some effect in animal studies and may warrant further investigation (112,114). Diverse other treatments such as barbiturates, hypothermia, prostacyclin, hyperosmolar agents, naloxone and steroids do not appear to have any sustained benefit.

Rheologic Therapy

Routine use of hemodilution has not been shown to be of consistent benefit in cerebral infarction (56,65). In cases of markedly elevated hematocrit in the setting of polycythemia vera or secondary polycythemia due to congenital heart disease the risk of cerebral infarction is increased and phlebotomy with fluid replacement with colloid or plasma may be necessary.

The use of pentoxifylline to decrease red blood cell deformability in acute nonhemorrhagic stroke was tested in 297 patients started within 12 hours of onset of symptoms (69). It was given initially intravenously, then orally for 25 days. It was found to be of no benefit.

Future Directions in Therapy for Cerebral Ischemia

Although a clear cut protocol for aggressive treatment of cerebral infarction has yet to be established; cerebral infarction is no longer to be treated by just rest and time. The therapies under investigation at the present time are based on an understanding of the cellular and hemodynamic pathophysiology of cerebral ischemia and infarction. New methods of prevention of cerebral infarction are now available with the goal of reducing its incidence. The optimal therapy for cerebral infarction will most likely be a "cocktail" in which drugs to decrease cellular ischemic damage will be combined with thrombolytic therapies. In the next few years results from trials ongoing at the present time will be revealed and new trials on new therapies are presently being organized. Cerebral infarction should soon be a "treatable disease."

REFERENCES

1.   Abbott, R.D., Y. Yin,D.M. Reed, K. Yano, Risk of stroke in male cigarette smokers. *N. Engl .J .Med* .315:717-720, 1986.

2.   Ackerman, R.H., J.A.Correia, N.A. Alpert et al: Positron emission tomography imaging in stroke using compounds labeled with oxygen-15. *Arch Neurol* 38:537-541,1981.

3.   Adams, H.P., N.F. Kassell, D.J. Boarini, G. Kongable, The clinical spectrum of aneurysmal subarachnoid hemorrhage. *J. Stroke Cerebrovasc. Dis.* 1:3-8,1991.

4.   Albers, G.W., M.P. Goldberg, D. Choi, N-methyl-D-aspartate antagonists: ready for clinical trial in brain ischemia? *Ann. Neurol.* 25:398-403,1989.

5.   Alberts, M.J., Genetic aspects of cerebrovascular disease. *Stroke* 22:276-280,1991.

6.   American Heart Association: 1992 Heart and Stroke Facts, Dallas 1991.

7.   The Asymptomatic Carotid Atherosclerosis Study Group: Study design for randomized prospective trial of carotid endarterectomy for asymptomatic atherosclerosis. *Stroke* 20:844-849,1989.

8.   Atlas, S.W., A.S. Mark, R.I. Grossman, J.M. Gomori, Intracranial hemorrhage: Gradient-echo MR imaging at 1.5T. *Radiology* 168:803-807, 1988.

9.   Bevan, H., K. Sharma, W. Bradley, Stroke in young adults. *Stroke* 21:382-386, 1990.

10.   The Boston Area Anticoagulation Trial for Atrial Fibrillation Investigators. The effect of low-dose warfarin on the risk of stroke in patients with nonrheumatic atrial fibrillation. *N. Engl. J. Med.* 323:1505-1511, 1990.

11.   Bougousslavsky, J., A. Delaloye-Bischof, F. Regli, B. Delaloye, Prolonged hypoperfusion and early stroke after transient ischemic attack. *Stroke* 21:40-46,1990.

12.   Bougousslavsky, J., F. Regli, Ischemic stroke in adults younger than 30 years of age. *Arch Neurol* 44: 479-485, 1987.

13.   Brey, R.L., RG. Hart, D.G. Sherman, C.H. Tegler, Antiphospholipid antibodies and cerebral ischemia in young people. *Neurology* 40:1190-1196,1990.

14.   Bridgers, S.L., G. Koch, C. Munera, N.M. Karwon Kurtz, Intravenous nimodipine in acute stroke: interim analysis of randomized trials. *Stroke* 22:153,1991.

15.   Brott, T., Thrombolytic therapy for stroke. *Cerebrovasc. Brain Metab. Rev.* 3:91-113,1991.

16.   Buchan, A.M., Do NMDA antagonists protect against cerebral ischemia: Are clinical trials warranted? Cerebrovasc. *Brain. Metab. Rev.* 2:1-26, 1990.

17.   Caplan, L., Stroke and drug abuse. *Stroke* 13:869-872, 1982.

18.   Carlberg, B., K. Asplund, E. Hagg, Factors influencing admission blood pressure levels in patients with acute stroke. *Stroke* 22:527-530, 1991.

19.   Carmargo, C.A., Moderate alcohol consumption and stroke: the epidemiologic evidence. *Stroke* 20:1611-1626, 1989.

20.   Cerebral Embolism Task Force: Cardiogenic brain embolism. *Arch. Neurol.* 43:71-84, 1986; 46:727-743, 1989.

21.   Chimowitz, M.I., J. Mancini, Asymptomatic coronary artery disease in patients with stroke: prevalence, prognosis, diagnosis, and treatment. *Stroke* 23: 433-436, 1992.

22.   Colditz, G.A., R. Bonita, M.J. Stampfer, W. Willett,B. Rosner , F.E. Speizer, Hennekens. Cigarette smoking and risk of stroke in middle-aged women. *N. Engl. J. Med.* 318:937-941, 1988.

23.   Collaborative Group for the Study of Stroke in Young Women: Oral contraceptives and stroke in young women. *JAMA* 231:718-722, 1975.

24.   Conomy, J.P., R.W. Kellermeyer, Delayed cerebrovascular consequences of therapeutic radiation. A clinicopathologic study of a stroke associated with radiation-related carotid arteriopathy. *Cancer* 36:1702-1708, 1975.

25.   Controversies in Neurology: Hypertension in acute ischemic strokes. *Arch. Neurol.* 42,999-1002, 1985.

26.   Controversies in Neurology: The secondary prevention of strokes in patients with atrial fibrillation. *Arch. Neurol.* 43:66-70, 1986.

27.   Cotman, C.W., L.L. Iversen, Excitatory amino acids in the brain-focus on NMDA receptors. *Trends Neurosci.* 10:263-265, 1987.

28.   Cujec, B., P. Polasek, C. Voll, A. Shuaib, Transesophageal echocariography in the detection of potential cardiac source of embolism in stroke patients. *Stroke* 22:727-733,1991.

29.   Daras, M., A.J. Tuchman, S. Marks, Central nervous system infarction related to cocaine abuse. *Stroke* 22:1320-1325,1991

30.   Del Zoppo, G.J.: Thrombolytic therapy in cerebrovascular disease. *Stroke* 23:7-12, 1988.

31. Devinsky, O., C.K. Petito, D.R. Alonso, Clinical and neuropathological findings in systemic lupus erythematosus: The role of vasculitis, heart emboli, and thrombotic thrombocytopenic purpura. *Ann. Neurol.* 23:380-384,1988.

32.   DeWitt, L.D., L.R. Wechsler, Transcranial Doppler. *Stroke* 19:915-921, 1988.

33.   Di Pasquale, G., A. Andreoli, G. Carini, M. Dondi, S. Urbinati, M. Ruffini, G. Pinelli, Noninvasive screening for silent ischemic heart disease in patients with cerebral ischemia: use of dipyridamole-thallium myocardial imaging. *Cerebrovasc. Dis.* 1:31-37,1991.

33a. Dyken, M.L., H.M.J. Barnett, J.D. Easton, et al., Low-dose aspirin and stroke - "It ain't mecessarily so". *Stroke* 23: 1395-1399, 1992.

34.   The EC/IC Bypass Study Group: Extracranial-intracranial arterial bypass surgery does not reduce the risk of ischemic stroke. *New Eng. J. Med.* 313:1191-1200, 1985.

35.   Engstrom, H.W. et al: Cerebral infarctions and transient neurologic deficits associated with acquired immunodeficiency syndrome. *Am. J. Med.* 86:528-532, 1989.

36.   European Carotid Surgery Trialist's Collaborative Group: MRC European Carotid Surgery Trial: Interim results for symptomatic patient's with severe (70-99%) or mild stenosis (0-29%) carotid stenosis. *Lancet* 337:1235-1243, 1991

37.   Fayad, P.B., L.M. Brass, Single photon emission computed tomography in cerebrovascular disease. *Stroke* 22:950-954,1991.

38.   Feldmann, E.: Intracerebral hemorrhage. *Stroke* 22:684-691,1991.

39.   Feussner, J.R., D.B. Matchar, When and how to study the carotid arteries. *Ann. Int. Med.* 109:805-818,1988.

40.   Fisher, M.: Atherosclerosis; cellular aspects and potential interventions. *Cerebrovasc. Brain. Metab. Rev.* 3:114-133, 1991.

41.   Frisoni, G.B., G.P. Anzola, Vertebrobasilar ischemia after neck motion. *Stroke* 22:1452-1460, 1991.

42.   Fuster, V. ,J.L. Halperin, Left ventricular thrombi and cerebral embolism. *N. Engl. J. Med.* 320:392, 1989.

43.   Futrell, N., C. Milikan, Frequency, etiology, and prevention of stroke in patients with systemic lupus erythematosus. *Stroke* 20:583-591,1989.

44.   Gardner, T.J., P.J. Horneffer, T.A. Manolio, et al: Stroke following coronary artery bypass grafting: a ten year study. *Ann. Thorac. Surg.* 40:574-581, 1985.

45.   Garraway, W.M., J.P. Whisnant, A.J. Furlan, et al: The declining incidence of stroke *N. Engl. J. Med.* 300:449, 1979.

46.   Gelmers, H.J., K. Gorter, C.J. DeWeerdt, et al: A controlled trial of nimodipine in acute ischemic stroke. *N. Engl. J. Med.* 318:203-207, 1988.

47.   Gent, M.: Single studies and overview analyses: is aspirin of value in cerebral ischemia? *Stroke* 18:541-544, 1987.

48.   Gent, M., J.A. Blakely, J.D. Easton, et al: The Canadian-American Ticlopidine Study in Thromboembolic Stroke: Design, organization and baseline results. *Stroke* 19:1203-1210, 1988.

49.   Gent, M., J.A. Blakely, V. Hachinski, et al: A secondary prevention, randomized trial of suloctidil in patients with a recent history of thromboembolic stroke. *Stroke* 16:416-424,1985.

50. Gent, M., J.A. Blakely, J. Easton, D.J. Ellis, V. Hachinski, V., et al: The Canadian American Ticlopidine Study (CATS) in thromboembolic stroke. *Lancet* 1:1215-1220, 1989.

51.   Gilman, S.: Neurological complications of open heart surgery. *Ann. Neurol.* 28:475-476,1990.

52.   Ginsberg, M.: Local metabolic responses to cerebral ischemia. *Cerebrovasc. Brain. Metab. Rev.* 2:58-93,1990.

53.   Giubilei, F., G.L. Lenzi, V. Di Piero, et al: Predictive value of brain perfusion single-photon emission computed tomography in acute ischemic stroke. *Stroke* 21:895-900,1990.

54.   Gorelick, P.B.: The status of alcohol as a risk factor for stroke. *Stroke* 20:1607-1610, 1989.

55.   Grant, E.G. et al: Cerebrovascular ultrasound imaging. *Rad. Clin. N. Am.* 26: 1111-1130, 1988.

56.   Grotta, J.C.: Current status of hemodilution in acute cerebral ischemia. *Stroke* 18:689-690, 1987.

57.   Hart, R.G., M.C. Kanter, Hematologic disorders and ischemic stroke. A selective review. *Stroke* 21;111-1121, 1990.

58.   Hass, W.K., J.D. Easton, H.P. Adams, et al.: A randomized trial comparing ticlopidine hydrochloride with aspirin for the prevention of stroke in high risk patients. *N. Eng .J. Med.* 321;501-507, 1989.

59.   Hakim, A.M., A. Ryder-Cooke, D. Melanson, Sequential computerized tomographic appearance. *Stroke* 14:893-7, 1983.

60.   Haley, E.C., N.F. Kassel, J.C. Torner, Failure of heparin to prevent progression in progressing ischemic infarction. *Stroke* 19:10, 1988.

61.   Hankey, G.: Isolated angiitis/angiopathy of the central nervous system. *Cerebrovasc. Dis.* 1:2-15,1991.

62.   Harrison, M.J.G.: Influence of hematocrit in the cerebral circulation. *Cerebrovasc. Brain. Metab. Rev.* 1:55-67, 1990

63.   Hass, W.: The cerebral ischemic cascade. *Neurol. Clin. North. Am.* 1:345, 1983.

64.   Heiss, W-D., V. Holthoff, G. Pawlik, M. Neveling, Effect of nimodipine on regional cerebral glucose metabolism in patients with acute ischemic stroke as measured by positron emission tomography. *J. Cereb. Blood. Flow. Metab.* 10:127-132,1990.

65.   Heros, R.C., K. Korosue, Hemodilution for cerebral ischemia. *Stroke* 20:423-427, 1989.

66.   Hess, D.C., J. Krauss, R.J. Adams, F.T. Nichols, D.I. Zhang, Rountree H.A.. Anticardiolipin antibodies: A study of frequency in TIA and stroke. *Neurology* 41:525-528,1991.

66a. Hobson, R.W., D.G. Weiss, W.S. Fields, et al., Efficacy of carotid endarterectomy for asymptomatic carotid stenosis, *N. Eng. J. Med* 328: 221-227, 1993

67. Holman, B.L., S.S. Tumeh, Single-photon emission computed tomography (SPECT). *JAMA* 263:561-564, 1990.

68. Horning, D.C., M. Kaps, Hacke, G. Kramer, O. Busse, F. Alchner, Nimodipine in acute ischemic stroke: results of the Nimodipine German Austrian Stroke Trial. *Stroke* 22:153,1991.

69. Hsu, C.Y., J.W. Norris,E.L. Hogan, et al: Pentoxifylline in acute nonhemorrhagic stroke: a randomized, placebo-controlled double-blind trial. *Stroke* 19:716-722, 1988.

70. Jamieson, D.G., A. Alavi, P. Jolles et al: Positron emission tomography in the investigation of central nervous system disorders. *Rad. Clin. N. Am.* 26:1075-1088, 1988.

71. Jenkins, A., D.M. Hadley,G.M. Teasdall, B. Condon, P. Macpherson, J. Patterson, MR imaging of acute subarachnoid hemorrhage. *J. Neurosurg.* 68:731-736, 1988.

72. Kido, D.K., R.J. Panzer, J. Szumowski, Hollander, et al: Clinical evaluation of stenosis of the carotid bifurcation with magnetic resonance angiographic techniques. *Arch. Neurol.* 48:484-489,1991.

73. Kertesz, A. , S.E. Black, L. Nicholson, T. Carr, The sensitivity of MRI in stroke. *Neurology* 37:1580-5, 1987.

74. Klag, M.J., P.K. Whelton, A.J. Seidler, Decline US stroke mortality: Demographic trends and antihypertensive treatment. *Stroke* 20:14, 1989.

75. Klein, G.M., T.P. Seland, Occlusive cerebrovascular disease in young adults. *Can. J. Neurol. Sci.* 11:302-304, 1984.

76. Krendel, D.A., S.M. Ditter, M.R. Frankel, W.K. Ross, Biopsy-proven cerebral vasculitis associated with cocaine abuse. *Neurology* 40,1092-1094,1990.

77. Kushner, M.J., Prospective study of anticardiolipin antibodies in stroke. *Stroke* 21: 295-298,1990.

78. Lee, R.J., T. Bartzokis, T-K Yeoh, H.R. Grogin, D. Choi, I. Schnittger, Enhanced detection of intracardiac sources of cerebral emboli by transesophageal echocardiography. *Stroke* 22:734-739,1991.

79.	Lenzi, G.L., R.S. Frackowiak, T. Jones, Regional cerebral blood flow, oxygen utilization, and oxygen extraction in acute hemispheric stroke. *J. Cereb. Blood Flow Metab.* 2:231-235, 1982.

80.	Levine. S.R., J.C. Brust, N. Futrell et al: Cerebrovascular complications of the use of the "crack" form of alkaloid cocaine. *New Eng. J. Med.* 323:699-704, 1990.

81.	Levine. M., J. Hirsh, Hemorrhagic complications of long-term anticoagulant therapy for ischemic cerebral vascular disease. *Stroke* 17:111-116, 1986.

82.	Love. B.B., J. Biller, M.P. Jones, H.P. Adams, A. Bruno, Cigarette smoking: a risk factor for cerebral infarction in young adults. *Arch. Neurol.* 47: 693-698,1990.

83.	Marie. C., J. Bralet, Blood glucose level and morphological brain damage following cerebral ischemia. *Cerebrovasc. Brain Metab. Rev.* 3:29-38, 1991.

84.	Martinez-Vila. E., F. Guilen, J. Villanueva et al: Placebo-controlled trial of nimodipine in the treatment of acute ischemic cerebral infarction. *Stroke* 21:1023-1028, 1990.

85.	Mauer. A.H.: Nuclear medicine: SPECT comparisons to PET. *Rad. Clin. N. Am.* 26:1059-1074, 1988.

86.	Meldrum. B.: Protection against ischaemic neuronal damage by drugs acting on excitatory neurotransmission. *Cerebrovasc. Brain Metab. Rev.* 2:27-57, 1990.

87.	Merz. B.: Large trial finds ticlopidine superior to aspirin in preventing stroke: Medical news and perspectives. *JAMA* 261:1541, 1989.

88.	Meyer. F.B., I. Meissner, N. Fode, T. Losasso, Carotid endarterectomy in elderly patients. *Mayo Clin Proc* 66:464-469,1991.

89.	Meyer. J.S., E. Stoica, I. Pascu, K. Shimazu, A. Hartmann, Catecholamine concentrations in CSF and plasma of patients with cerebral infarction and hemorrhage. *Brain* 96:277-288,1973.

90.	Mokri. B.: Traumatic and spontaneous extracranial internal carotid artery dissections. *J. Neurol.* 237:356-361,1990.

91.	Moody. D.M., M.A. Bell, V.R. Challa, W.E. Johnston, D.S. Prough, Brain microemboli during cardiac surgery or aortography. *Ann. Neurol.* 28:447-486,1990.

92.   Myers. M.G., J.W. Norris, V.C. Hachinski, M.J. Sole, Plasma norepinephrine in stroke. *Stroke* 12:200-203, 1981.

93.   Newell. D.W., S. Grady, Sirotta, H.R. Winn, Evaluation of brain death using transcranial Doppler. *Neurosurgery* 24:509-513,1989.

94.   North American Symptomatic Carotid Endarterectomy Trial Collaborators. Beneficial effect of carotid endarterectomy in symptomatic partients with high-grade stenosis. *N. Engl. J. Med.* 325:445-53, 1991.

95.   North American Symptomatic Carotid Endarterectomy Trial (NASCET) Steering Committee. North American Symptomatic Carotid Endarterectomy Trial: Methods, patient characteristics, and progress. *Stroke* 22:711-720,1991.

96.   Natowicz. M., R.I. Kelly, Mendelian etiologies of stroke. *Ann. Neurol.* 22:175-192, 1987.

97.   Oleson. J.: Cerebral and extracranial circulatory disturbances in migraine: pathophysiological implications. *Cerebrovasc. Brain Metab. Rev.* 3:1-28,1991.

98.   Petersen. P., G. Boysen, J. Godtfredsen, E.D. Andersen, B. Andersen, Placebo-controlled, randomized trial of warfarin and aspirin for prevention of thromboembolic complications of chronic atrial fibrillation. *Lancet* 1:175-179, 1989.

99.   Petty,   G.W., D. O. Wiebers, I. Meissner, Transcranial Doppler ultrasonography: clinical applications in cerebrovascular disease. *Mayo Clin Proc* 65:1350-1364,1990.

100.   Powers, W.J.: Cerebral hemodynamics in ischemic cerebrovascular disease. *Ann. Neurol.* 29:231-240,1991.

101.   Pulsinelli, W.A., D.E. Levy, B. Sigsbee, P. Scherer, F. Plum, Increased damage after ischemic stroke in patients with hyperglycemia with or without established diabetes mellitus. *Am. J. Med.* 74:540-544,1983.

102.   Ramadan, N.M., R. Deveshwar, S.R. Levine, Magnetic resonance and clinical cerebrovascular disease. *Stroke* 20:1279-1283, 1989.

103.   The rt-PA / Acute Stroke Study Group: An open safety/efficacy trial of rt-PA in acute thromboembolic stroke: final report. *Stroke* 22:153, 1991.

104.   Report of the American Academy of Neurology, Theraputics and Technology Assessment Subcommittee. Interim assessment: Carotid endarterectomy. *Neurology* 40:682-683, 1990.

105. Robinson, M.J.. G.M. Teasdale, G.M.: Calcium channel antagonists in the management of subarachnoid hemorrhage. *Cerebrovasc. Brain Metab. Rev.* 2:205-226, 1990.

106. Rosenbaum, D., J. Zabramski, J. Frey, F. Yatsu, J. Marler, R. Spetzler, J. Grotta, Early treatment of ischemic stroke with a calcium antagonist. *Stroke* 22:437-441,1991.

107. Ross, J.S., T.J. Masaryk, M.T. Modic, P.M. Ruggieri, E.M. Haacke, W.R. Selman, Intracranial aneurysms: evaluation by MR angiography. *AJNR* 11:449-455,1990.

108. Rothman ,S.M., J.W. Olney, Excitotxicity and the NMDA receptor. *Trends Neurosci* 10:299-302, 1987.

109. Salgado, A.V.: Central nervous system complications of infective endocarditis. *Stroke* 22:1461-1463, 1991

110. Scatton, B., C. Carter, J. Benavides, C. Giroux, N-methyl-D-aspartate receptor antagonists: A novel therapeutic perspective for the treatment of ischemic brain injury. *Cerebrovasc Dis.* 1: 121-135, 1992.

111. Scheinberg ,P.: Heparin anticoagulation. *Stroke* 20:173, 1989.

111a. Schöning, M., R. Buchholz, J. Walter, Comparative study of transcranial color duplex sonography and transcranial Doppler sonography in adults. *J. Neurosurg* 78: 776-784, 1993.

112. Schmidley, J.W.: Free radicals in central nervous system ischemia. *Stroke* 21:1086-1090, 1990.

113. Siesjo, B.K.: Historical overview. Calcium, ischemia, and death of brain cells. *Ann NY Acad Sci* 522: 638-661, 1988.

114. Siejo, B.K., C.D. Agardh, F. Bengtsson, Free radicals and brain damage. *Cerebrovasc. Brain Metab. Rev.* 1:165-211, 1989.

115. Simon, R.P., J.H. Swan, T. Griffiths et al. Blockade of N-methyl D-aspartate receptors may protect against ischemic damage. *Science* 226: 850-852, 1984.

116. Skinhoj Olsen, T.: Should induced hypertension or hypotension ever be used in the treatment of stroke? *Acta. Med. Scand. Suppl.* 678:113-120, 1983.

117. Sloan, M.A.: Thrombolysis and stroke: Past and future. *Arch. Neurol.* 44:748, 1987.

118. Special Report From the World Health Organization: Stroke-1989: Recommendations on stroke prevention, diagnosis, and therapy. *Stroke* 20:1407-1431, 1989.

119. Special Report From the National Institute of Neurologic Disorders and Stroke. Classification of cerebrovascular disease III. *Stroke* 21;637-676, 1990.

120. Spence, J.D., R.F. Del Maestro, Hypertension in acute ischemic strokes: Treat. *Arch. Neurol.* 42:1000-1002, 1985.

121. Stroke Prevention in Atrial Fibrillation Study Group Investigators. Preliminary report of the stroke prevention in atrial fibrillation study. *New Eng. J. Med.* 322:863-868, 1990.

121a. Stroke Prevention in Atrial Fibrillation Investigators: Stroke prevention in atrial fibrillation study: final results. *Circulation* 84: 527-539, 1991.

121b. The Stroke Prevention in Atrial Fibrillation Investigators: Predictors of thromboembolism in atrial fibrillation. Clinical features of patients at risk. *Ann. Int. Med.* 116: 1-5, 1992.

122. Sze, P.C., Reitman, D., Pincus, M.M., Sacks, H.S., Chalmers, T.C.: Antiplatelet agents in the secondary prevention of stroke: meta-analysis of the randomized control trials. *Stroke* 19:436-442,1988.

123. Tegler, C.H., T.R. Downes, Cardiac imaging in stroke. *Stroke* 22:1206-1211, 1991.

124. Trust Study Group. Randomized, double-blind, placebo controlled trial of nimodipine in acute stroke. *Lancet* 336:1205-1209, 1990.

125. Wallace, J.D., L.L. Levy, Blood pressure after stroke. *JAMA* 246:2177, 1981.

126. Wechsler et al: Transcranial doppler in cerebrovascular disease. *Stroke* 17:905-912, 1986.

127. Weibers, D.O.: Ischemic cerebrovascular complications of pregnancy. *Arch. Neurol.* 42: 1106-1113, 1985.

128. Williams, S.R., H.A. Crockard, D.G. Gadian, Cerebral ischemia studied by nuclear magnetic resonance spectroscopy. *Cerebrovasc. Brain Metab. Rev.* 1:91-114,1989.

129. Wise, R.J., S. Bernardi,N.J. Frackowiak et al: Serial observation in the pathophysiology of acute stroke. *Brain* 106:197-200, 1983.

130. Wolf, P.A., R.B. D'Angostino, W.B. Kannel, R. Bonita, A.J. Belanger, Cigarette smoking as a risk for stroke. *JAMA* 259:1025-1029, 1988.

131. Wong, M.C.W., E.C. Haley, E.C.: Calcium antagonists: Stroke therapy coming of age. *Stroke* 21:494-501, 1990.

132. Woo, J., C.W.K. Lam, R. Kay,A.H.Y. Wong ,R. Teoh, M.G. Nicholls, The influence of hyperglycemia and diabetes mellitus on immediate and three month morbidity and mortality after acute stroke. *Arch. Neurol.* 47:1174-1177, 1990.

133. Yatsu, F.M., R.G. Hart, J.P. Mohr, J.C. Grotta, Anticoagulation of embolic strokes of cardiac origin. *Neurology* 38:314-316,1988.

134. Yatsu, F.M., J.P. Mohr, Anticoagulation therapy for cardiogenic emboli to brain. *Neurology* 32:274, 1982.

135. Zivin, J., M. Fisher, U. DeGirolami et al: Tissue plasminogen activator reduces neurologic damage after cerebral embolism. *Science* 230:1289, 1985.

136. Zivin, J., V. Mazzarella, Tissue plasminogen activator plus glutamate antagonist improves outcome after embolic stroke. *Arch Neurol* 48: 1235-1238, 1991.

5

GUIDELINES FOR ANESTHESIA AND CEREBRAL PROTECTION IN NEUROVASCULAR SURGERY

Woodrow Wm. Wendling, M.D., Ph.D.
Assistant Professor of Anesthesiology
Temple University Hospital
Philadelphia, PA 19140

Christer Carlsson, M.D., Ph.D.
Professor of Anesthesiology and Physiology
Temple University Hospital and School of Medicine
Philadelphia, PA 19140

INTRODUCTION

The administration of anesthesia for a neurovascular procedure is not "straight forward." Anesthetic agents, mode of ventilation and physiologic variables all have effects on the cerebral circulation, and may very well have significant effects on areas of borderline perfusion during the procedure. Carotid arteries or major cerebral vessels may be deliberately or inadvertently occluded for a short period of time, either during extracranial procedures (such as carotid endarterectomy) or intracranial procedures (such as clipping of an intracranial aneurysm). At such times cerebral protection becomes an important issue. The purpose of this chapter is to first discuss cerebral ischemia, neuroanesthesia, and cerebral protection in general, and then to give guidelines for anesthesia for specific neurovascular procedures.

CEREBRAL ISCHEMIA

The brain has virtually no energy stores and meets its energy requirements almost exclusively by oxidative metabolism of glucose which is continuously delivered with the blood. Therefore, even short periods of decreased cerebral blood flow can result in insufficient supplies of both oxygen and glucose, and put the brain at risk for injury (1-3).

Cerebral ischemia is a reduction of cerebral blood flow to levels that are insufficient to maintain normal function, metabolism and integrity. The critical reduction can be defined as various degrees of **incomplete ischemia** as well as **complete ischemia**. From an anatomic point of view the ischemia can be **global** or **focal**. It is important to understand the differences between these categories, since they show differences in intracellular metabolic events. The extent of cerebral injury is determined not only by the duration and type of ischemia, but also by other factors such as brain temperature, type of anesthesia, nutritional status, and circumstances during the period of recirculation.

It is well known that cerebral blood flow (CBF) is autoregulated within the normal range of the blood pressure. When mean arterial pressure falls below 60-70 mm Hg, autoregulation fails and blood flow passively follows the blood pressure. When CBF falls below 25% of normal the electrical activity of the brain ceases (4). A further drop in CBF to below 10% of normal leads to membrane failure and deterioration of energy balances (5-6) and triggers reactions leading to irreversible neuronal damage (5).

Following total interruption of CBF an almost immediate cessation of mitochondrial adenosine triphosphate (ATP) production takes place. The anaerobic breakdown of glucose results in an accumulation of lactate and a metabolic acidosis. In studies in rats complete ischemia reduced ATP stores to about 10% after 3 minutes (7). Lactate accumulation in the brain is determined by pre-ischemic levels of glucose and glycogen (8). In the study by Ljunggren et al (7) maximal levels of tissue lactate were found to be 12-13 micromoles/gram. In a model of incomplete ischemia the constant supply of glucose led to even higher lactate levels-up to 30 micromoles/gram (9).

Complete ischemia leads to influx of calcium and sodium ions into the cells and an efflux of potassium (10,11). Furthermore, excitatory amino acid transmitters such as glutamate are released (12). According to the excitotoxic hypothesis of brain injury, glutamate is released during cerebral ischemia and causes excessive excitation at N-methyl-D-aspartate (NMDA) receptors (13). This excitation leads to excessive influx of sodium and water, which causes acute damage, and calcium, which causes delayed and more permanent damage (13). Interaction of receptor transmitters and elevation of intracellular calcium in combination with decreased energy stores lead to catabolic reactions (14,15) such as lipolysis and proteolysis, which have also been suggested to be important factors in the development of neuronal damage (16).

The period after the ischemic insult has been studied since it has been shown to have a biphasic blood flow pattern. Initially hyperemia is found, this being important since it may improve neurophysiologic parameters even after very long ischemia (17). However, the period of hyperemia is then often followed by decreased cerebral blood flow, the so-called "no-reflow" phenomenon (18). It has in fact been suggested that most of ischemic cell damage occurs during this period.

GENERAL PRINCIPLES OF NEUROANESTHESIA

The most common type of general anesthesia today is "balanced anesthesia", meaning that several drugs are given to the patient. Anesthesia is typically induced with a short-acting intravenous agent such as sodium thiopental and maintained with combinations of volatile inhalational anesthetics (such as isoflurane), nitrous oxide, benzodiazepines (such as midazolam) and narcotics (such as fentanyl), along with non-depolarizing neuromuscular junction blockers for muscle relaxation. Each of the anesthetic agents has effects on cerebral circulation and metabolism (19-26); the effects from combinations of them are less known.

Drugs that increase cerebral blood flow are not necessarily beneficial and those that decrease the flow are not necessarily detrimental. An increase in CBF increases intracranial volume and thus causes intracranial pressure (ICP) to rise, especially if ICP is already elevated. Conversely, drugs that reduce CBF may cause a fall in ICP, creating more space in the cranial vault and more room for the neurosurgeon, so-called "brain relaxation."

The following summary of the effects of common anesthetic agents on CBF and metabolism assumes a familiarity with the main features of cerebral metabolism (27).

As a general rule, all inhalational anesthetics in current use **increase** CBF to some extent; the rank order is halothane >> enflurane > isoflurane > nitrous oxide. The potent volatile inhalational anesthetics in clinical use-isoflurane, enflurane, and halothane-all produce a dose-related reduction in the cerebral metabolic rate (CMR) while simultaneously causing cerebral vasodilatation (28-32). Accordingly, the volatile agents are said to "uncouple" flow and metabolism. Halothane causes the most cerebral vasodilatation (30-31); it is rarely used in adults in the USA because of the risk of hepatotoxicity. Enflurane in high concentrations can induce seizures, particularly in combination with hyperventilation and hypocapnia (23,33). Of the three volatile agents isoflurane produces the least increase in CBF, and accordingly is used more often in neuroanesthesia.

For a long period of time nitrous oxide was felt to be inert, but now a vast number of direct studies in animals and indirect studies in man show that nitrous oxide produces a significant rise in CBF (25,26,34-37). The rise in CBF with nitrous oxide is probably more pronounced initially and then declines over time. The human studies (36,37) showed that nitrous oxide elevated intracranial pressure, as would be expected for an agent that increased CBF.

Most intravenous anesthetics **decrease** CBF, except for ketamine (38). The barbiturates produce a dose-related decrease in CBF and CMR (22,39,40); flow and metabolism are "coupled." With the barbiturates, the maximal reduction in CMR occurs with the dose producing an isoelectric electroencephalogram (EEG); the CMR is reduced to about 40-50% of normal (39,40). Barbiturates reduce only one component of cerebral metabolic activity, neuronal electro-physiologic activity, but have little effect on energy utilization to maintain cellular homeostasis (41).

Etomidate, a non-barbiturate anesthetic agent, also produces a decrease in CMR (42-44) and suppresses EEG activity (44-49); however, etomidate differs from the barbiturates in several important aspects. Etomidate is a potent direct cerebral vasoconstrictor, independent of its effects on CMR (43). The pattern of metabolic depression produced by etomidate differs markedly from that produced by barbiturates; etomidate decreases cerebral glucose consumption in some, but not all cerebral structures, and the effects on $CMR_{glucose}$ are not dose-dependent (50). Etomidate has been associated with seizures in humans and with EEG spike and wave activity (51-54).

Unlike most intravenous anesthetics, ketamine increases CBF (38,55). The mechanism by which ketamine produces cerebral vasodilatation is unclear. Ketamine may increase CBF by increasing CMR; however, the increases in CMR repeatedly observed in animals have not been verified in humans (38,55-58). Ketamine may also increase CBF by directly dilating the cerebral vasculature (59).

The potent narcotic analgesics, such as fentanyl and sufentanil, reduce CBF and CMR, but may at very high concentrations produce seizure-like EEG activity and an increase in CBF (24,60-61). The use of sufentanil in neuroanesthesia is somewhat controversial, because of reports that this narcotic increased cerebrospinal fluid pressure in humans with supratentorial tumors (62) and CBF in dogs (63). On the other hand, more recent studies found sufentanil to have no significant effect on CBF (64), ICP (65) or brain retractor pressure (66) in humans.

The "balanced anesthetic" technique used for neuroanesthesia today involves combinations of several drugs, which together could produce different alterations in cerebral blood flow and metabolism. It is very unlikely, however, that any combination of drugs could reduce the overall metabolism by more than 50-60%, a level reached when the EEG becomes isoelectric (28,29,67).

CEREBRAL PROTECTION

Protection of the brain during various ischemic events has been of great interest for many decades, and has been intensively studied during the last two. Kety and Schmidts' pioneering measurements of CBF and cerebral oxygen consumption (68) were only the beginning of our understanding that these parameters varied with the state of consciousness, and that anesthetic agents might be useful since they reduced metabolic demand. Unfortunately, results of cerebral ischemia studies have been less positive than promised or expected, and no striking protective method has been found by using anesthetic agents.

The only method of cerebral protection that is used routinely during surgical procedures is intentional hypothermia during cardiopulmonary bypass. Experimentally and clinically, the hypothermic brain tolerates a low-flow or a no-flow situation longer than the normothermic brain (69). Hypothermia strikingly decreases metabolism and does so in direct relationship to the temperature achieved (69). A reduction in body temperature by 1°C will reduce CBF and $CMRO_2$ by 5-7% (69-72), meaning that a fall in temperature by 10°C will reduce cerebral metabolism by ≥50% (69), a significant figure and fully equivalent to deep barbiturate anesthesia. Unlike the barbiturates, hypothermia reduces **both** neuronal electrophysiologic activity and the activity associated with maintenance of cellular homeostasis (41,69).

Recent investigations indicate that even mild hypothermia has a substantial protective effect against ischemic injury (73-77). At 35°C, a temperature producing only a 10-15% reduction in $CMRO_2$ (70), there was almost total protection in a rat model of cerebral ischemia (78). Mild hypothermia (31-34°C) improves neurologic outcome even when initiated immediately after the ischemic insult (79-82). These findings suggest that reduced metabolic demand is not the only mechanism of hypothermic cerebral protection, and that other mechanisms must be involved (83). Mild hypothermia can block the release of glutamate that occurs with ischemia (74), and thus may prevent excitotoxic tissue injury.

Of all the anesthetic agents, the barbiturates have been most extensively investigated for their cerebral protective effects. In animal models, high doses of barbiturate (thiopental or pentobarbital) decrease the neurologic deficit and mortality from cerebral infarction induced by middle cerebral artery occlusion (84-88). The barbiturate must be administered before, during, or just after the ischemic event in order to demonstrate a protective effect (89-90), and the maximal protective effect occurs at doses that produce an isoelectric EEG (91).

The barbiturates have been utilized for intraoperative cerebral protection in humans undergoing various procedures, including carotid endarterectomy (92-96), clipping of intracranial aneurysms (97-99), and cardiac surgery (100-103). However, only two prospective randomized studies have been obtained with barbiturates in humans, and only one of these studies showed cerebral protection (100). Thiopental decreased neuropsychiatric complications after open heart procedures with normothermic cardiopulmonary bypass (CPB) (100), but not after coronary artery bypass graft procedures with hypothermic CPB (101).

Etomidate has recently been used as a "cerebral protectant" in humans undergoing clipping of intracranial aneurysms (104-106), but this use is controversial (107,108). Etomidate, like thiopental, decreases CMR (42-44) and suppresses EEG activity (44-49), but has less cardiovascular depression (e.g., hypotension) and more rapid emergence from anesthesia. Etomidate has been assessed for a cerebral protective effect in incomplete cerebral ischemia in three studies on rats (54,108,109). In one study, low-dose (0.02 mg/kg/min i.v.) etomidate reduced neurologic deficits and mortality, but high-dose (0.2 mg/kg/min i.v.) etomidate was associated with a worse outcome despite a similar reduction in $CMRO_2$ (54). In the other studies, etomidate sufficient to produce burst suppression resulted in a significant reduction of histologic injury in the hippocampus but not in other structures (108). Further studies, in particular investigations that compare the efficacy of etomidate and barbiturates "head to head," are needed to determine if etomidate is as effective a cerebral protectant as thiopental (107,109).

Anesthetic agents that decrease CMR and produce an isoelectric EEG should **not** be assumed to be cerebroprotective. Propofol, a short-acting intravenous anesthetic, and isoflurane both produce CMR and EEG suppression like the barbiturates (29,110), and yet do not appear to provide the same cerebral protective benefits (83,111). Most animal models of cerebral ischemia, except one by Milde and coworkers (112), fail to demonstrate a cerebral protective effect for isoflurane (78,83,107).

Certain anesthetic agents may be cerebroprotective without decreasing $CMRO_2$. For example, ketamine has no demonstrable effect on $CMRO_2$ or $CMR_{glucose}$ in humans (38), and causes both increases and decreases in regional $CMR_{glucose}$ in animal models (55-58). Ketamine and another N-methyl-D-aspartate (NMDA) receptor antagonist, dizocilpine, have been shown to be cerebral protective in some (113-116) but not all (81,117,118) animal models of cerebral ischemia. Ketamine may protect the brain in ischemia, not by reducing cerebral metabolic demand, but by blocking the excitotoxic action of glutamate at NMDA receptors (13).

ANESTHETIC GUIDELINES FOR CAROTID ARTERY SURGERY

Anesthesia for carotid artery surgery has three primary goals: to protect the heart from ischemia, to protect the brain from ischemia, and to have the patient awaken quickly after the operation (119).

From a cardiac standpoint, the goal of anesthesia is to maintain normal hemodynamics, oxygenation, and ventilation. It is important to avoid those factors which decrease myocardial oxygen supply (i.e., decrease coronary blood flow or oxygen delivery) or increase myocardial oxygen demand-tachycardia, volume overload, hypotension or hypertension, extreme hypocapnia, hypoxia, extreme anemia, or coronary spasm (120). A high percentage of carotid end-arterectomy candidates have advanced or severe coronary artery disease, even those with no history or electrocardiographic evidence of heart disease (121).

The second goal of anesthesia during carotid endarterectomy is to protect the brain from ischemia (119). The guidelines to attain this goal are to maintain a normal or high normal blood pressure, maintain normocarbia or slight hypocarbia, maintain normoglycemia, monitor for cerebral perfusion, and treat cerebral ischemia if it occurs.

A normal or high normal blood pressure is desirable to preserve collateral flow to the brain during carotid occlusion (119,122). If cerebral autoregulation is impaired in areas of the brain threatened by ischemia, then blood flow passively follows systemic arterial blood pressure in these regions (123). One technique to increase cerebral blood flow to these regions is to deliberately induce mild hypertension with a phenylephrine infusion. This deliberate hypertension is not without risk, however, as it may also increase cardiac workload and precipitate cardiac ischemia (124). Larson (125) has recommended that deliberate hypertension be avoided in patients with known cardiac disease and in those who develop electrocardiographic ST segment depression as hypertension is induced.

The optimal arterial carbon dioxide tension ($PaCO_2$) for carotid artery surgery is controversial, though most anesthesiologists now opt for slight hypocarbia or normocarbia (119,122,125). Slight hypocarbia may possibly divert cerebral blood flow to potentially ischemic areas of brain by constricting normal non-ischemic vessels.

Glucose-containing intravenous solutions should not be used in any circumstance in which there is a risk of a cerebral ischemic event and in which there is not a specific indication for glucose administration (107,126). Lactated Ringer's solution should also be avoided, since lactate is metabolized to glucose (119). Hyperglycemia is associated with worse neurologic outcome in some but not all animal models of focal cerebral ischemia (127-130). The increased cerebral injury with glucose administration may be related to anaerobic lactic acid production.

There are many ways to assess for cerebral perfusion during carotid artery surgery, including unprocessed and processed EEGs, somatosensory evoked potentials (SSEPs), carotid artery stump pressure, xenon[133] measurement of regional cerebral blood flow (rCBF), and an awake neurologic assessment during regional anesthesia. These different methods to monitor for cerebral dysfunction have **not** been shown to improve patient outcome (131). However, logic dictates that monitoring techniques assuring adequate cerebral function at the lowest myocardial work should have a place in carotid endarterectomy surgery (131).

If cerebral ischemia occurs during clamping of the carotid artery, as evidenced by a "significant" EEG change (greater than 50% reduction in amplitude or flattening of the EEG or SSEP), a stump pressure less than 50 mm Hg, or a clamped rCBF less than 20 cc/min per 100 g brain, then the neurosurgeon may selectively shunt the carotid artery (132,133). Shunting during carotid endarterectomy is controversial, however, and some surgeons either shunt routinely or shunt very rarely (132). The advantage of the shunt is that it preserves carotid flow, while potential risks include thromboembolism, intimal dissection, thrombus formation, air embolism, and obstruction of the surgical field (134).

A second method to treat for cerebral ischemia, should it be detected during carotid endarterectomy, is to use a barbiturate such as thiopental to induce pharmacologic cerebral protection (92-96). Large quantities of thiopental (10-25 mg/kg body weight) are needed to produce an EEG pattern of burst suppression (less than 6 bursts of EEG activity per minute), and additional increments of thiopental are often needed to maintain burst suppression (95). A single prophylactic bolus of thiopental does not protect against prolonged cerebral ischemia (135,136).

The final goal of anesthesia for carotid endarterectomy is to have the patient awaken quickly at the end of the procedure. This post-operative goal is most influenced by the preoperative choice of premedication and the intraoperative choice of anesthesia. The goal of premedication is to prevent anxiety-induced tachycardia and hypertension, but to avoid oversedation resulting in preoperative hypoxia and hypercarbia and in delayed postoperative awakening (137). If thiopental is administered for cerebral protection, then awakening from anesthesia will be delayed. When Hicks and coworkers (95) used thiopental for cerebral protection during carotid endarterectomy, the patients all required 1/2 to 3 hours to become fully responsive, and 12 of 77 patients required postoperative ventilatory support for up to one hour.

ANESTHESIA FOR INTRACRANIAL
NEUROVASCULAR SURGERY

In patients with subarachnoid hemorrhage (SAH) due to a ruptured intracranial aneurysm, the main therapeutic goals are to maintain an adequate cerebral perfusion pressure (CPP) and to prevent recurrent hemorrhage. It is important to maintain an adequate CPP, because the SAH patient often has impaired autoregulation, decreased carbon dioxide responsiveness of cerebral vessels, abnormalities of regional CBF, and increased intracranial pressure (ICP) (138). A large number of these patients will go on to develop delayed cerebral vasospasm several days after the initial hemorrhage (139,140). Since CPP is equal to mean arterial pressure (MAP) minus ICP, CPP can be increased either by increasing MAP or decreasing ICP. However, these same maneuvers also increase the transmural pressure across the wall of the aneurysm and thus predispose the aneurysm to rupture and rebleed (138).

To a large extent, the preoperative management of the patient with an intracranial aneurysm depends on the severity of the SAH. In patients with good neurologic function (i.e., a favorable Hunt-Hess grade of I or II) (141), several maneuvers are employed, mostly to prevent further hemorrhage before surgery. These maneuvers include bed rest, light sedation with benzodiazepines, stool softeners to prevent straining, antihypertensive therapy, and antifibrinolytic agents such as epsilon aminocaproic acid or tranxemic acid. Unfortunately, these maneuvers are all "double-edged" swords with the potential for benefit or risk. Cerebroselective calcium entry blockers such as nimodipine are employed to reduce the occurrence of severe neurologic deficits due to cerebral arterial vasospasm (142-145).

Patients with poor or deteriorating function (i.e., with Hunt-Hess grades of III to V) due to increasing ICP or vasospasm require more aggressive monitoring (arterial catheterization, central venous or Swan-Ganz catheterization, ICP monitoring) and therapy (controlled hyperventilation, mannitol, steroids) in an intensive care setting. In patients with good neurologic function, such monitoring and therapy might not be instituted until the time of surgery.

The two main therapeutic goals in the patient with aneurysmal SAH, to maintain an adequate CPP and to prevent recurrent hemorrhage, continue through surgery. There are several additional "common sense" aims for anesthetic management-to avoid hypoxia, extreme anemia, hypercarbia, hyperthermia, extreme hyperglycemia, and sudden hyper- or hypotension, and to facilitate surgical access to the aneurysm.

Hypercarbia must be avoided because it markedly increases CBF and ICP. Normocarbic or slightly hypocarbic ($PaCO_2$ = 35) hyperventilation is desirable in patients with favorable Hunt-Hess grades of I to II. In patients with Hunt-Hess grades of III to V due to SAH, hypocapnic hyperventilation to a $PaCO_2$ of 25-30 may be necessary to decrease ICP and intracranial volume (146-148) and to facilitate surgical exposure of the aneurysm.

Hyperthermia should be avoided because it increases $CMRO_2$ and CBF, and worsens histologic outcome after ischemia in animal experiments (76). Normothermia is a reasonable goal. Some institutions employ mild hypothermia (33-34°C) for aneurysm clipping procedures (107), because of the cerebroprotective effect noted in animal models of ischemia (73-77). Practices for achieving intraoperative hypothermia and for rewarming vary between institutions (107). Most problems with mild hypothermia occur during rewarming to normothermia-delayed awakening, undesirable cardiovascular effects (hypertension and tachycardia), and shivering.

Normoglycemia is desirable during intracranial neurovascular procedures, and insulin administration to achieve plasma glucose concentrations less than 150 mg/dl would appear to be appropriate (107). Elevated plasma glucose levels increase brain damage during ischemia (127,128,149). There are even experimental studies suggesting "protective" effects from lowered glucose levels (150-152). These provocative findings go against basic medical knowledge, as the brain is dependent on glucose for its metabolism.

The challenge for the anesthesiologist is to provide adequate anesthesia with hemodynamic stability, and in addition to avoid sudden changes in blood pressure. Hypertension, whether a consequence of preoperative anxiety, coughing, endotracheal intubation during induction of anesthesia, or surgical stimulation, increases transmural pressure across the wall of the aneurysm and can cause rebleeding. On the other hand, severe hypotension decreases CPP. Potential causes of hypotension include volume depletion, venous air emboli, and intraoperative hemorrhage from the aneurysm.

Two techniques to facilitate surgical access to the aneurysm are to decrease intracranial volume and to intentionally induce hypotension. Decreasing intracranial volume-with diuretics (mannitol and furosemide), steroids (dexamethasone), hyperventilation, barbiturates, and other anesthetic agents-minimizes brain retraction and tissue injury (153,154). Controlled hypotension (to a CPP of 50-60 mm Hg) reduces transmural pressure across the wall of the aneurysm, making it softer and more pliable (138). Also, if the aneurysm ruptures, blood loss is decreased and bleeding is easier to control.

If pharmacologic cerebral protection is required during clipping of an intracerebral aneurysm, the barbiturate thiopental is the most reasonable choice at the present time. Thiopental has several advantages: (1) It decreases intracranial volume (by decreasing $CMRO_2$ and CBF); (2) It reduces transmural pressure across the aneurysmal wall (by producing hypotension); (3) Thiopental has proven to be cerebroprotective in animal models of focal ischemia (84-88) and in one controlled human study (100); (4) It has previously been employed as a cerebral protective agent during aneurysm clipping (97-99). The raw EEG should be monitored intraoperatively to document that EEG burst suppression is attained and maintained. Unfortunately, high doses of thiopental are required to produce burst suppression (95,100), which can cause untoward hypotension during the procedure and will delay emergence from anesthesia in the immediate postoperative period.

SUMMARY

In the future new modalities or drugs will be suggested for cerebral protection. Before "cerebroprotective" agents are used in general practice, however, they must be tested in small animal models, in primates, and in very well controlled clinical studies. It is of no value to use drugs or combinations of drugs that may only have theoretical benefits, before they are of proven efficacy. Such an approach will only confuse the "cerebral protection" field. In general practice, the best advice is to know the pharmacologic effects of common drugs, and to use each drug within its therapeutic range.

ACKNOWLEDGEMENTS

The writing of this review article was supported in part by Biomedical Research Support Grant SO7 RR05417 from the Division of Research Resources, National Institute of Health. Dr. Wendling is the recipient of an Anesthesiology Young Investigator Award from the Foundation for Anesthesia Education and Research and Janssen Pharmaceutica.

REFERENCES

1.   Lowry, O.H., J.V. Passonneau, F.X. Hasselberger, D.W. Schultz, Effect of ischemia on known substances and cofactors of the glycolytic pathway in brain. *J. Biol. Chem.*, 1964; 239: 18-30

2.   Goldberg, N.D., J.V. Passonneau, O.H. Lowry, Effects of changes in brain metabolism on the level of citric acid cycle intermediates. *J. Biol. Chem.*, 1966; 241: 3997-4003

3.   Silver, I.A.: Changes in PO_2 and ion fluxes in cerebral hypoxia-ischemia. In: *Tissue hypoxia and ischemia*. M. Reivich, ed. Plenum Press, New York, 1977: 299-312

4.   Branston, N.M., L. Symon, H.A. Crockard, E. Pazztor, Relationships between the cortical evoked potential and local cortical blood flow following acute middle cerebral artery occlusion in the baboon. *Exp. Neurol.*, 1974; 45: 195-208

5.   Astrup, J., L. Symon, N.M. Branston, N.A. Lassen, Cortical evoked potential and extracellular K+ and H+ at critical levels of brain ischemia. *Stroke*, 1977; 8: 51-57

6.   Branston, N.M., A.J. Strong, L. Symon, Extracellular potassium activity, evoked potential and tissue blood flow. Relationships during progressive ischemia in baboon cerebral cortex. *J. Neurol. Sci.*, 1977; 32: 305-321

7.   Ljunggren, B., H. Schutz, B.K. Siesjo, Changes in energy state and ischemic parameters of the rat brain during complete compression ischemia. *Brain Res.*, 1974; 73: 277-289

8.   Gatfield, P.D., O.H. Lowry, D.W. Schultz, J.V. Passonneau, Regional energy reserves in mouse brain and changes with ischemia and anesthesia. J. *Neurochem.*, 1966; 13: 185-195

9.   Nordstrom, C.H., B.K. Siesjo, Effects of phenobarbital in cerebral ischemia. Part I. Cerebral energy metabolism during incomplete ischemia. *Stroke*, 1978; 9: 327-335

10.   Hansen, A.J., T. Zeuthen, Extracellular ion concentrations during spreading depression and ischemia in the rat brain cortex. *Acta Physiol. Scand.*, 81; 113: 437-445

11.   Harris, R.J., L. Symon, N.M. Branston, M. Bayhan, Changes in extracellular calcium activity in cerebral ischemia. *J. Cereb. Blood Flow Metab.*, 1981; 1: 203-209

12. Beneviste, H., J. Drejer, A. Schousboe, N.H. Diemer, Elevation of the extracellular concentrations of glutamate and aspartate in rat hippocampus during transient cerebral ischemia monitored by intracerebral microdialysis. *J. Neurochem.*, 1984; 43: 1369-1374

13. Collins, R.C., B.H. Dobkin, D.W. Choi, Selective vulnerability of the brain: New insights into the pathophysiology of stroke. *Ann. Intern. Med.*, 1989; 110: 992-1000

14. Yoshida, S., T. Inoh, K. Sano, M. Kubota, H. Shimazaki, N. Ueta, Effect of transient ischemia on free fatty acids and phospholipids in gerbil brain. Lipid peroxidation as possible cause of postischemic injury. *J. Neurosurg.*, 1980; 53: 323-331

15. Rehncrona, S., E. Westerberg, B. Akesson, B.K. Siesjo, Brain cortical fatty acids and phospholipids during and following complete and severe incomplete ischemia. *J. Neurochem.*, 1982; 38: 84-93

16. Siesjo, B.K., T. Wieloch, Cerebral metabolism in ischemia: Neurochemical basis for therapy. *Br. J. Anaesth.*, 1985; 57: 47-62

17. Hossman, K.A, H. Lechtape-Gruter, V. Hossman, The role of cerebral blood flow for the recovery of the brain after prolonged ischemia. *Z. Neurol.*, 1973; 204: 281-299

18. White, B.C., J.G. Wiegenstein, C.D. Winegar, Brain ischemic anoxia. *JAMA*, 1984; 251: 1586-1590

19. Carlsson, C., M. Hagerdal, A.E. Kaasik, B.K. Siesjo, The effects of diazepam on cerebral blood flow and oxygen consumption in rats and its synergistic interaction with nitrous oxide. *Anesthesiology*, 1976; 45: 319-325

20. Nilsson, L.: The influence of barbiturate anesthesia upon the energy state and upon acid-base parameters of the brain in arterial hypotension and in asphyxia. *Acta Neurol. Scand.*, 1971; 47: 233-253

21. Carlsson, C., J. Harp, B.K. Siesjo, Metabolic changes in the cerebral cortex of the rat induced by intravenous "Pentothalsodium." *Acta Anaesthesiol. Scand. Suppl.*, 1975; 57: 7-17

22. Nilsson, L., B.K. Siesjo, The effect of phenobarbitone anesthesia on blood flow and oxygen consumption in the rat brain. *Acta Anaesthesiol. Scand. Suppl.*, 1975; 57: 18-24

23. Michenfelder, J.D., R.F. Cucciara, Canine cerebral oxygen consumption during enflurane anesthesia and its modification during induced seizures. *Anesthesiology*, 1974; 41: 231-236

24.   Carlsson, C., D.S. Smith, M.M. Keykhah, J.R. Harp, The effects of high dose fentanyl on cerebral circulation and metabolism in rats. *Anesthesiology,* 1982; 57: 375-380

25.   Baughman, V.L., W.E. Hoffman, D.J. Miletich, R.F. Albrecht, Cerebrovascular and metabolic effects of N_2O in unrestrained rats. *Anesthesiology,* 1990; 73: 269-272

26.   Carlsson, C., U.S. Vasthare, R.F. Tuma, M. Rocco, R. Dombkoski, Influence of nitrous oxide administration and discontinuation thereof on blood flow in cerebral cortex, cerebellum and brain stem in the rat. *Acta Anaesthesiol. Scand.,* 1991; 35: 771-775

27.   Siesjo, B.K.: Brain energy metabolism. Wiley and Sons: Chichester, New York, Brisbane, and Toronto, 1978.

28.   Michenfelder, J.D., R.A. Theye, In vivo toxic effects of halothane on canine cerebral metabolic pathways. *Amer. J. Physiol.,* 1975; 229: 1050-1055

29.   Newberg, L.A., J.H. Milde, J.D. Michenfelder, The cerebral metabolic effects of isoflurane at and above concentrations that suppress cortical electrical activity. *Anesthesiology,* 1983; 59: 23-28

30.   Todd, M.M., J.C. Drummond, A comparison of the cerebral vascular and metabolic effects of halothane and isoflurane in the cat. *Anesthesiology,* 1984; 60: 276-282

31.   Eintrei, C., W. Leszniewski, C. Carlsson, Local application of [133]Xenon for measurement of regional blood flow (rCBF) during halothane, enflurane, and isoflurane anesthesia in humans. *Anesthesiology,* 1985; 63: 391-394

32.   Newman, B., A.W. Gelb, A.M. Lam, The effect of isoflurane-induced hypotension on cerebral blood flow and cerebral metabolic rate for oxygen in humans. *Anesthesiology,* 1986; 644: 307-310

33.   Neigh, J.L., J.K. Garman, J.R. Harp, The electroencephalographic pattern during anesthesia with ethrane. *Anesthesiology,* 1971; 35: 482-487

34.   Sakabe, T., T. Kuramoto, S. Inoue, H. Takeshita, Cerebral effects of nitrous oxide in the dog. *Anesthesiology,* 1978; 48: 195-200

35.   Pellegrino, D.A., D.J. Miletich, W.E. Hoffman, R.F. Albrecht, Nitrous oxide markedly increases cerebral cortical metabolic rate and blood flow in the goat. *Anesthesiology,* 1984; 60: 405-412

36.   Henriksen, H.T., P.B. Jorgensen, The effect of nitrous oxide on intracranial pressure in patients with intracranial disorders. *Br. J. Anaesth.*, 1973; 45: 486-492

37.   Sakabe, T., T. Kuramoto, S. Kumakae, H. Takeshita, Cerebral response to the addition of nitrous oxide to halothane in man. *Br. J. Anaesth.*, 1976; 48: 957-962

38.   Takeshita, H.,Y. Okuda, A. Sari, The effects of ketamine on cerebral circulation and metabolism in man. *Anesthesiology*, 1972; 36: 69-75

39.   Pierce, E.C., Jr., C.J. Lambertsen, S. Deutsch, P.E. Chase, H.W. Linde, R.P. Dripps, H.L. Price, Cerebral circulation and metabolism during thiopental anesthesia and hyperventilation in man. *J. Clin. Invest.*, 1962; 41, 1664-1671

40.   Michenfelder, J.D.: The interdependency of cerebral functional and metabolic effects following massive doses of thiopental in the dog. *Anesthesiology*, 1974; 41: 231-236

41.   Drummond, J.C., H.M. Shapiro, Cerebral physiology. Miller, R.D. (Ed.): Anesthesia, 3rd. Ed. Churchill Livingstone, New York, 1990: 621-658

42.   Renou, A.M., J. Vernhiet, P. Macrez, P. Constant, J. Billerey, M.Y. Khadaroo, J.M. Caille, Cerebral blood flow and metabolism during etomidate anesthesia in man. *Br. J. Anaesth.*, 1978; 50: 1047-1051

43.   Milde, L.N., J.H. Milde, J.D. Michenfelder, Cerebral functional, metabolic, and hemodynamic effects of etomidate in dogs. *Anesthesiology*, 1985; 63: 371-377

44.   Cold, G.E., V. Eskesen, H. Eriksen, B.B. Lyon, Changes in $CMRO_2$, EEG and concentration of etomidate in serum and brain tissue during craniotomy with continuous etomidate supplemented with N_2O and fentanyl. *Acta Anesthesiol. Scand.*, 1986; 30: 159-163

45.   Doenicke, A., J. Kugler, G. Penzel, M. Laub, L. Kalmar, I. Killian, H. Bezecny, Cerebral function under etomidate, a new non-barbiturate i.v. hypnotic. *Anaesthesist*, 1973; 22: 357-366

46.   Ghoneim, M.M., T. Yamada, Etomidate: a clinical and electroencephalo-graphic comparison with thiopental. *Anaesthesiol. Analg.*, 1977: 56: 479-485

47.   Doenicke, A., B. Loffler, J. Kugler, H. Suttmann, B. Grote, Plasma concentration and EEG after various regimens of etomidate. *Br. J. Anaesth.*, 1982: 54: 393-400

48.   Freye, E., E. Hartung, A. Klatte, J. Abel, Plasma levels of alfentanil and etomidate and their relation to compressed power spectral analysis of the EEG. *Acta Anaesthesiol. Belg.*, 1983; 34: 87-96

49.   Schuttler, J., H. Schwilden, H. Stoeckel, Infusion strategies to investigate the pharmacokinetics and pharmacodynamics of hypnotic drugs: etomidate as an example. *Eur. J. Anaesthesiol.*, 1985; 2: 133-142

50.   Davis, D.W., A.M. Mans, J.F. Biebuyck, R.A. Hawkins, Regional brain glucose utilization during etomidate anesthesia. *Anesthesiology*, 1986; 64: 751-757

51.   Ebrahim, Z.Y., G.E. DeBoer, H. Luders, J.F. Hahn, R.P. Lesser, Effect of etomidate on the encephalogram of patients with epilepsy. *Anaesthesiol. Analg.*, 1986; 65: 1004-1006

52.   Gancher, S., K.D. Laxer, W. Krieger, Activation of epileptogenic activity by etomidate. *Anesthesiology*, 1984; 61: 616-618

53.   Grant, I.S., G. Hutchinson, Epileptiform seizures during prolonged etomidate sedation. *Lancet* II: 511-512, 1983

54.   Baughman, V.L., W.E. Hoffman, D.J. Miletich, R.F. Albrecht, Cerebral metabolic depression and brain protection produced by midazolam and etomidate in the rat. *J. Neurosurg. Anesthesiol.*, 1989; 1: 22-28

55.   Dawson, B., J.D. Michenfelder, R.A. Theye, Effects of ketamine on canine cerebral blood flow and metabolism: Modification by prior administration of thiopental. *Anaesthesiol. Analg.*, 1971; 50: 443-447
56.   Crosby, G., A.M. Crane, L. Sokoloff, Local changes in cerebral glucose utilization during ketamine anesthesia. *Anesthesiology*, 1982; 56: 437-443

57.   Cavazzuti, M., C.A. Porro, G.P. Biral, C. Benassi, G.C. Barbieri, Ketamine effects on local cerebral blood flow and metabolism in the rat. *J. Cereb. Blood Flow Metab.*, 1987; 7: 806-811

58.   Davis, D.W., A.M. Mans, J.F. Biebuyck, R.A. Hawkins, The influence of ketamine on regional brain glucose use. *Anesthesiology*, 1988; 69: 199-205

59.   Fukuda, S., T. Murakawa, H. Takeshita, N. Toda, Direct effects of ketamine on isolated canine cerebral and mesenteric arteries. *Anaesthesiol. Analg.*, 1983; 62: 553-558

60.   Michenfelder, J.D., R.A. Theye, Effects of fentanyl, droperidol, and "Innovar" on canine cerebral metabolism and blood flow. *Br. J. Anaesthesiol.*, 1971; 43: 630-635

61.   Keykhah, M.M., D.S. Smith, C. Carlsson, Y. Safo, I. Englebach, J.R. Harp, Influence of sufentanil on cerebral metabolism and circulation in the rat. *Anesthesiology*, 1985; 63: 274-277

62.   Marx, W., N. Shah, C. Long, E. Arbit, J. Galicich, C. Mascott, K. Mallya, R. Bedford, Sufentanil, alfentanil, and fentanyl: Impact on cerebrospinal fluid pressure in patients with brain tumors. *J. Neurosurg. Anesthesiol.*, 1989; 1: 3-7

63.   Milde, L.N., J.H. Milde, W.J. Gallagher, Effects of sufentanil on cerebral circulation and metabolism in dogs. *Anaesthesiol. Analg.*, 1990; 70: 138-146

64.   Mayer, N., C. Weinstabl, I. Podreka, C.K. Spiss, Sufentanil does not increase cerebral blood flow in healthy human volunteers. *Anesthesiology*, 1990; 73: 240-243

65.   Weinstabl, C., N. Mayer, B. Richling, T. Czech, C.K. Spiss, Effect of sufentanil on intracranial pressure in neurosurgical patients. *Anesthesia*, 1991; 46: 837-840

66.   Herrick, I.A., A.W. Gelb, P.H. Manninen, H. Reichman, S. Lownie, Effects of fentanyl, sufentanil, and alfentanil on brain retractor pressure. *Anaesthesiol. Analg.*, 1991; 72: 359-363

67.   Michenfelder, J.D.: In vivo effects of massive concentrations of anesthetics on canine cerebral metabolism. Fink, B.R. (Ed.): Molecular mechanisms of anesthesia. Raven Press, New York, 1975: 537-561

68.   Kety, S.S., C.F. Schmidt, The determination of cerebral blood flow in man by the use of nitrous oxide in low concentrations. *Amer. J. Physiol.*, 1945; 143: 53-66

69.   Michenfelder, J.D.: Anesthesia and the brain. Churchill Livingstone, New York, 1988

70.   Hagerdal, M., J.R. Harp, L. Nilsson, B.K. Siesjo, The effect of induced hypothermia upon oxygen consumption in the rat brain. *J. Neurochem.*, 1975; 24: 311-316

71. Carlsson, C., M. Hagerdal, B.K. Siesjo, The effect of hyperthermia upon oxygen consumption and upon organic phosphates, glycolytic metabolites, citric acid cycle intermediates and associated amino acids in the rat cerebral cortex. *J. Neurochem.*, 1976; 26: 1001-1006

72. Michenfelder, J.D., R.A.Theye, Hypothermia: effect on canine brain and whole-body metabolism. *Anesthesiology*, 1968; 29: 1107-1112

73. Busto, R., W.D. Deitrich, M.Y.-T. Globus , I. Valdes, P. Scheinberg, M.D. Ginsburg, Small differences in intraischemic brain temperature critically determine the extent of ischemic neuronal injury. *J. Cereb. Blood Flow Metab.*, 1987; 7: 729-738

74. Busto, R., M. Y.-T. Globus, D. Dietrich, E. Martinez, I. Valdes, M.D. Ginsberg, Effect of mild hypothermia on ischemia-induced release of neuro-transmitters and free fatty acids in the brain. *Stroke*, 1989; 20: 904-910

75. Minamisawa, H., C.-H. Nordstrom, M.-L. Smith, B.K. Siesjo, The influence of mild body and brain hypothermia on ischemic brain damage. *J. Cereb. Blood Flow Metab.*, 1990; 10: 365-374

76. Minamisawa, H., M. Smith, B.K. Siesjo, The effect of mild hyperthermia and hypothermia on brain damage following 5, 10, and 15 minutes of forebrain ischemia. *Ann. Neurol.*, 1990; 28: 26-33

77. Welsh, F.A., R.E. Sims, V.A. Harris, Mild hypothermia prevents ischemic injury in gerbil hippocampus. *J. Cereb. Blood Flow Metab.*, 1990; 10: 557-563

78. Sano, T., J.C. Drummond, P.M. Patel, M.R. Grafe, J.C. Watson, D.J. Cole, A comparison of the cerebral protective effects of isoflurane and mild hypothermia in a model of incomplete forebrain ischemia in the rat. *Anesthesiology*, 1992; 76: 221-228

79. Boris-Moller, F., M. Smith, B.K. Siesjo, Effects of hypothermia on ischemic brain damage: a comparison between preischemic and postischemic cooling. *Neurosci. Res. Commun.*, 1989; 5: 87-94

80. Busto, R., D. Dietrich, M.Y.-T. Globus, M.D. Ginsberg, Postischemic moderate hypothermia inhibits CA1 hippocampal ischemic neuronal injury. *Neurosci. Lett.*, 1989; 101: 299-304

81. Buchan, A., W.A. Pulsinelli, Hypothermia but not the N-methyl-D-aspartate antagonist, MK-801, attenuates neuronal damage in gerbils subjected to transient global ischemia. *J. Neurosci.*, 1990; 10: 311-316

82.   Hoffman, W.E., C. Werner, V.L. Baughman, C. Thomas, D.J. Miletich, R.F. Albrecht, Postischemic treatment with hypothermia improves outcome from incomplete cerebral ischemia in rats. *J. Neurosurg. Anaesthesiol.*, 1991; 3: 34-38

83.   Todd, M., D.S. Warner, A comfortable hypothesis reevaluated: Cerebral metabolic depression and brain protection during ischemia. *Anesthesiology*, 1992; 76: 161-164

84.   Smith, A.L., J.T. Hoff, S.L. Nielsen, C.P. Larson, Barbiturate protection in acute focal cerebral ischemia. *Stroke*, 1974; 5: 1-7

85.   Hoff, J.T., A.L. Smith, H.L. Hankinson, S.L. Nielsen, Barbiturate protection from cerebral infarction in primates. *Stroke*, 1975; 6: 28-33

86.   Michenfelder, J.D., J.H. Milde, Influence of anesthetics on metabolic, functional and pathological responses to regional cerebral ischemia. *Stroke*, 1975; 6: 405-410

87.   Michenfelder, J.D., J.H. Milde, T.M. Sundt, Cerebral protection by barbiturate anesthesia. *Arch. Neurol.*, 1976; 33: 345-350

88.   Corkill, G., S. Sivalingam, J.A. Reitan, A. Gilroy, M.G. Helphrey, Dose dependency of the post-insult protective effect of pentobarbital in the canine experimental stroke model. *Stroke*, 1978; 9: 10-12

89.   Corkill, G., O.K. Chikovani, I. McLeish, L.W. McDonald, J.R. Youmans, Timing of pentobarbital administration for brain protection in experimental stroke. *Surg. Neurol.*, 1976; 5: 147-149

90.   Selman, W.R., R.F. Spetzler, R.A. Roski, U. Roessmann, R. Crumrine, R. Macko, Barbiturate coma in focal cerebral ischemia: Relationship of protection to timing of therapy. *J. Neurosurg.*, 1982; 56: 685-690

91.   Kassell, N.F., P.W. Hitchon, M.K. Gerk, M.D. Sokoll, T.R. Hill, Alterations in cerebral blood flow, oxygen metabolism, and electrical activity produced by high dose sodium pentothal. *Neurosurgery*, 1980; 7: 598-603

92.   Gross, C.E., H.P. Adams Jr., M.D. Sokoll, T. Yamada, Use of anticoagulants, electroencephalographic monitoring, and barbiturate cerebral protection in carotid endarterectomy. *Neurosurgery*, 1981; 9: 1-5

93.   Markowitz, I.P., M.F. Adinolfi, M.D. Kerstein, Barbiturate therapy in the postoperative endarterectomy patient with a neurologic deficit. *Am. J. Surg.*, 1984; 148: 221-223

94. McMeniman, W.J., J.P. Fletcher, J.M. Little, Experience with barbiturate therapy for cerebral protection during carotid endarterectomy. *Ann. R. Coll. Surg. Engl.*, 1984; 66: 361-364

95. Hicks, R.G., D.R. Kerr, D.A. Horton, Thiopentone cerebral protection under EEG control during carotid endarterectomy. *Anaesth. Intensive Care*, 1986; 14: 22-28

96. Spetzler, R.F., N. Martin, M.N. Hadley, R.A. Thompson, E. Wilkinson, P.A. Raudzens, Microsurgical endarterectomy under barbiturate protection; a prospective study. *J. Neurosurg.*, 1986; 65: 63-73

97. Sokoll, M.D., N.F. Kassell, L.R. Davies, Large dose thiopental for intracranial aneurysm surgery. *Neurosurgery*, 1982; 10: 555-562

98. Sokoll, M.D., N.F. Kassell, S.D. Gergis, Hemodynamic effects of N_2O, O_2 barbiturate anesthesia and induced hypotension in early versus late aneurysm clipping. *Neurosurgery*, 1982; 11: 352-355

99. Bendtsen, A.O., G.E. Cold, J. Astrup, J. Rosenorn, Thiopental loading during controlled hypotension for intracranial aneurysm surgery. *Acta Anaesthesiol. Scand.*, 1984; 28: 473-477

100. Nussmeyer, N.A., C. Arlund, S. Slogoff, Neuropsychiatric complications after cardiopulmonary bypass: Cerebral protection by a barbiturate. *Anesthesiology*, 1986; 64: 165-170

101. Zaidan, J.R., A. Klochany, W.M. Martin, J.S. Ziegler, D.M. Harless, R.B. Andrews, Effect of thiopental on neurologic outcome following coronary artery bypass grafting. *Anesthesiology*, 1991; 74: 406-411

102. Scheller, M.S.: Routine barbiturate brain protection during cardiopulmonary bypass cannot be recommended. *J. Neurosurg. Anesthesiol.*, 1992; 4: 60-63

103. Schell, R.M., J.G. Reves, Cerebral protection during cardiac surgery: Ban the barbiturates? *J. Neurosurg. Anesthesiol.*, 1992; 4: 64-67

104. Batjer, H.H., A.I. Frankfurt, P.D. Purdy, S.S. Smith, D.S. Samson, Use of etomidate, temporary arterial occlusion, and intraoperative angiography in surgical treatment of large and giant cerebral aneurysms. *J. Neurosurg.*, 1988; 68: 234-240

105. Muizelaar, J.P.: The use of electroencephalography and brain protection during operation for basilar aneurysms. *Neurosurgery*, 1989; 25: 899-903

106.   Rosenwasser, R.H., D.F. Jimenez, W.W. Wendling, C. Carlsson, Routine use of etomidate and temporary vessel occlusion during aneurysm surgery. *Neurological Res.*, 1991; 13: 224-228

107.   Drummond, J.C.: Cerebral ischemia: State of the art management. IARS Review Course Lectures, *Anesth. Analg.* (Suppl.), 1992; 120-128

108.   Watson, J.C., J.C. Drummond, P.M. Patel, T. Sano, W. Akrawi, U. Hoi Sang,   An assessment of the cerebral protective effects of etomidate in a model of incomplete forebrain ischemia in the rat. *Neurosurgery*, 1992; 30: 540-544

109.   Sano, T., P.M. Patel, J.C. Drummond, D.J. Cole, A comparison of the cerebral protective effects of etomidate, thiopental, and isoflurane in a model of forebrain ischemia in the rat. *Anesth. Analg.*, 1993; 76: 990-997

110.   Dam, M., C. Ori, G. Pizzolato, G. Ricchieri, A. Pellegrini, G. Giron, L. Battistin, L.: The effects of propofol anesthesia on local cerebral glucose utilization in the rat. *Anesthesiology*, 1990; 73: 499-505

111.   Ridenour, T.R., D.S. Warner, M.M. Todd, T.X. Gionet, Comparative effects of propofol and halothane on outcome from temporary middle cerebral artery occlusion in the rat. *Anesthesiology*, 1992; 76: 807-812

112.   Milde, L.N., J.H. Milde, W.L. Lanier, J.D. Michenfelder, Comparison of the effects of isoflurane and thiopental on neurologic outcome and neuropathology after temporary focal cerebral ischemia in primates. *Anesthesiology*, 1988; 69: 905-913

113.   Church, J., S. Zeman, D. Lodge, The neuroprotective action of ketamine and MK-801 after transient cerebral ischemia in rats. *Anesthesiology*, 1988; 69: 702-709

114.   Boxer, P.A., J.J. Cordon, M.E. Mann, L.C. Rodolosi, M.G. Vartanian, D.M. Rock, C.P. Taylor, F.W. Marcoux, Comparison of phenytoin with noncompetitive N-methyl-D-aspartate antagonists in a model of focal brain ischemia in rat. *Stroke*, 1990; 21 (Suppl. III): III-47-III-51

115.   Meyer, F.B., R.E. Anderson,   Friedrich, P.F.: MK-801 attenuates capillary bed compression and hypoperfusion following incomplete focal cerebral ischemia. *J. Cereb. Blood Flow Metab.*, 1990; 10: 895-902

116.   Hoffman, W.E., D. Pelligrino, C. Werner, E. Kochs, R.F. Albrecht, J. Esch, J. Sam, Ketamine decreases plasma catecholamines and improves outcome from incomplete cerebral ischemia in rats. *Anesthesiology*, 1992; 76: 755-762

117. Jensen, M.L., R.N. Auer, Ketamine fails to protect against ischaemic neuronal necrosis in the rat. *Br. J. Anaesth.*, 1988; 61: 206-210

118. Nellgard, B., I. Gustafson, T. Wieloch, T.: Lack of protection by the N-methyl-D-aspartate receptor blocker dizocilpine (MK-801) after transient severe cerebral ischemia in the rat. *Anesthesiology*, 1991; 75: 279-287

119. Roizen, M.F.: Anesthesia for vascular surgery. Barash, P.G., Cullen, B.F., Stoelting, R.K. (Eds.): Clinical Anesthesia. J.B. Lippincott Co., New York, 1989: 1015-1047

120. Thys, D.M., J.A. Kaplan, Cardiovascular physiology. Miller RD (Ed.): Anesthesia, 3rd. Ed. Churchill Livingstone, New York, 1990: 551-583

121. Sirna, S., J. Biller, D.J. Skorton, J.E. Seabold, Cardiac evaluation of the patient with stroke. *Stroke*, 1990; 21: 14-23

122. Ehrenfeld,W.K., W.K. Hamilton, C.P. Larson, Jr., R.F. Hickey, J.W. Severinghaus, Effect of CO_2 and systemic hypertension on downstream cerebral arterial pressure during carotid endarterectomy. *Surgery*, 1970; 67: 87-96

123. Michenfelder, J.D.: Anesthesia and surgery for cerebrovascular insufficiency: One approach at the Mayo Clinic. Roizen, M.F. (ed.): Anesthesia for Vascular Surgery. Churchill Livingstone, New York, 1990: 123-133

124. Smith, J.S., M.F. Roizen, M.K. Cahalan, D.J. Benefiel, P.N. Beaupre, Y.J. Sohn, B.F. Byrd, N.B. Schiller, R.J. Stoney, B.F. Ehrenfeld, J.E. Ellis, S. Aronson, Does anesthetic technique make a difference? Augmentation of systolic blood pressure during carotid endarterectomy: Effects of phenylephrine versus light anesthesia and of isoflurane versus halothane on the incidence of myocardial ischemia. *Anesthesiology*, 1988; 69: 846-853

125. Larson, C.P., Jr.: Anesthesia and surgery for cerebrovascular insufficiency: one approach at Stanford. Roizen, M.F. (Ed.): Anesthesia for Vascular Surgery. Churchill Livingstone, New York, 1990: 135-145

126. Sieber, F.E., D.S. Smith, R.J. Traystman, H. Wollman, Glucose: A reevaluation of its intraoperative use. *Anesthesiology*, 1987; 67: 72-81

127. Pulsinelli, W.A., S. Waldman, D. Rawlinson, F. Plum, Moderate hyperglycemia augments ischemic brain damage: a neuropathologic study in the rat. *Neurology*, 1982; 32: 1239-1246

128. Nedergaard, M.: Transient focal ischemia in hyperglycemic rats is associated with increased cerebral infarction. *Brain Res.*, 1987; 408: 79-85

129. Ginsberg, M.D., R. Prado, W.D. Dietrich, R. Busto, B.D. Watson, Hyperglycemia reduces the extent of cerebral infarction in rats. *Stroke*, 1987; 18: 570-574

130. Prough, D.S., A.T. Rogers, W.E. Johnston, Cardiopulmonary bypass and the brain. Intl. Anaesthesiol. Res. Soc. Refresher Course Lectures, 1992; 6-14

131. Roizen, M.F.: Anesthetic goals for operations to relieve or prevent cerebrovascular insufficiency. Roizen, M.F. (Ed.): Anesthesia for Vascular Surgery. Churchill Livingstone, New York, 1990: 103-122

132. Ferguson, G.G.: Carotid endarterectomy: To shunt or not to shunt? *Arch. Neurol.*, 1986; 43: 615-617

133. Lam, A.A.M., P.H. Manninen, G.G. Ferguson, W. Nantau, Monitoring electrophysiologic function during carotid endarterectomy-a comparison of somatosensory evoked-potentials and conventional electroencephalogram. *Anesthesiology*, 1991; 75: 15-21

134. Youngberg, J.A.: Perioperative anesthetic considerations for the patient for carotid artery surgery. Barash, P.G. (Ed.): ASA Refresher Courses in Anesthesiology, Vol. 15. J.B. Lippincott Co., Philadelphia, 1987: 209-220

135. Moffat, J.A., M.J. McDougall, D. Brunet, F. Saunders, E.S. Shelley, F.W. Cervenko, B. Milne, Thiopental bolus during carotid endarterectomy-rational therapy? *Can. Anaesth. Soc. J.*, 1983; 30: 615-622

136. Gelb, A.W., P. Floyd, P. Lok, S.J. Peerless, M. Farrell, A prophylactic bolus of thiopentone does not protect against prolonged focal cerebral ischaemia. *Can. Anaesthesiol. Soc. J.*, 1986; 33: 173-177

137. Clark, N.J., T.H. Stanley, Anesthesia for vascular surgery. Miller, R.D. (Ed.): Anesthesia, 3rd. Ed. Churchill Livingstone, New York, 1990: 1693-1736

138. Gelb, A.W., P. Newfield, Intracranial aneurysms. Matjasko J, Katz J (eds.): Clinical Controversies in Neuroanesthesia and Neurosurgery. Grune and Stratton, Inc., Orlando, FL, 1986; 33-256

139. Kassell, N.F., C.G. Drake, Timing of aneurysm surgery. *Neurosurgery*, 1982; 10: 514-519

140. Kassell, N.F., T. Sasaki, A.R.T. Colohan, G. Nazar , Cerebral vasospasm following aneurysmal subarachnoid hemorrhage. *Stroke*, 1986; 16: 562-572

141. Hunt, W.E., R.M. Hess, Surgical risk as related to time of intervention in the repair of intracranial aneurysms. *J. Neurosurg.*, 1968; 28: 14-20

142. Allen, G.S., H.S. Ahn, T.J. Preziosi, R. Battye, S.C. Boone, S.N. Chou, D.L. Kelly, B.K. Weir, R.A. Crabbe, P.J. Lavik, S.B. Rosenbloom, F.C. Dorsey, C.R. Ingram, D.E. Mellits, L.A. Bertsch, D.P.J. Boisvert, M.B. Hundley, R.K. Johnson, J.A. Strom, C.R. Transou, Cerebral arterial spasm-a controlled trial of nimodipine in patients with subarachnoid hemorrhage. *N. Engl. J. Med.*, 1983; 308: 619-624

143. Philippon, J., R. Grob, F. Dagreou, M. Guggiari, M. Rivierez, P. Viars, Prevention of vasospasm in subarachnoid hemorrhage. A controlled study with nimodipine. *Acta Neurochir. (Wien)*, 1986; 82: 110-114

144. Petruk, K.C., M. West, G. Mohr, B.K. Weir, B.G. Benoit, F. Gentili, L.B. Disney, M.I. Khan, M. Grace, R.O. Holness, M.S. Karwon, R.M. Ford, G.S. Cameron, W.S. Tucker, G.B. Purves, J.D.R. Miller, K.M. Hunter, M.T. Richard, F.A. Durity, R. Chan, L.J. Clein, F.B. Maroun, A. Godon: Nimodipine treatment in poor-grade aneurysm patients. Results of a multicenter double-blind placebo-controlled trial. *J. Neurosurg.*, 1988; 68: 505-517

145. Pickard, J.D., G.D. Murray, R. Illingworth, M.D.M. Shaw, G.M. Teasdale, P.M. Foy, P.R.D. Humphrey, D.A. Lang, R. Nelson, P. Richards, J. Sinar, S. Bailey, A. Skene, Effect of oral nimodipine on cerebral infarction and outcome after subarachnoid hemorrhage: British aneurysm nimodipine trial. *Br. Med. J.*, 1989; 298: 636-642

146. Kety, S.S., C.F. Schmidt, The effects of active and passive hyperventilation on cerebral blood flow, cerebral oxygen consumption, cardiac output and blood pressure of normal young men. *J. Clin. Invest.*, 1946; 25, 107-119

147. Kety, S.S., C.F. Schmidt, The effect of altered arterial tensions of carbon dioxide and oxygen on cerebral blood flow and cerebral oxygen consumption of normal young men. *J. Clin. Invest.*, 1948; 27: 484-491

148. Eklof, B., N.A. Lassen, L. Nilsson, K. Norberg, B.K. Siesjo, Blood flow and metabolic rate for oxygen in the cerebral cortex of the rat. *Acta Physiol. Scand.*, 1973; 88: 587-589

149. Lanier, W.L., K.J. Stangland, B.W. Scheithauer, J. Milde, J.D. Michenfelder, The effects of dextrose infusion and head position on neurologic outcome after complete cerebral ischemia in primates: examination of a model. *Anesthesiology*, 1987; 66: 39-48

150. Fukuoka, S., H. Yeh, T. Mandybur, J.M. Tew, Jr., Effect of insulin on acute experimental cerebral ischemia in gerbils. *Stroke*, 1989; 20: 396-399

151.   Voll, C.L., R.N. Auer,   The effect of postischemic blood glucose levels on ischemic brain damage in the rat. *Ann. Neurol.*, 1988; 24: 638-646

152.   LeMay, D.R., L. Gehua, G.B. Zelenock, L.G. D'Alecey,   Insulin administration protects neurologic function in cerebral ischemia in rats. *Stroke*, 1988; 19: 1411-1419

153.   Albin, M.S., L. Bunegin, M. Dujovny, M.H. Bennett, P.J. Jannetta, H.M. Wisotzkey,   Brain retraction pressure during intracranial procedures. *Surg. Forum*, 1975; 26: 499-500

154.   Rosenorn, J., N. Diemer,   The risk of cerebral damage during graded brain retractor pressure in the rat. *J. Neurosurg.*, 1985; 63: 608-611

6

CRITICAL CARE MANAGEMENT
OF NEUROVASCULAR PROBLEMS
IN PATIENTS UNDERGOING
NON-NEUROSURGICAL PROCEDURES

Christer Carlsson, M.D., Ph.D.

Professor of Anesthesiology and Physiology
Temple University Hospital and School of Medicine
Philadelphia, PA 19140

Woodrow Wm. Wendling, M.D., Ph.D.

Assistant Professor of Anesthesiology
Temple University Hospital
Philadelphia, PA 19140

INTRODUCTION

Medicine and surgery today encounter problems more difficult than before. Patients who are admitted for elective surgical procedures often have unrelated neurologic problems. This makes great demands on both the surgeon and the anesthesiologist to do a careful workup and to choose safe techniques in order to accomplish a successful outcome.

This chapter will discuss the relationship between neurological conditions and unrelated surgical procedures and will give some recommendations on how to plan in complex situations. Before further discussion, and without going into detail on cerebral blood flow regulation, cerebral metabolism maintenance or alterations (see previous chapters), the following brief summary will provide an introduction to the problems.

Regulation of cerebral blood flow (CBF) is complex and probably not fully understood. What we do know is that many factors--mean arterial blood pressure (MABP), temperature, arterial carbon dioxide content ($PaCO_2$), arterial oxygen content (PaO_2), hemoglobin, pH, intra- and extracellular potassium balance, and sympathetic nervous tone--are all involved. The CBF stays within very narrow limits so long as homeostasis is unperturbed. In humans the normal CBF is about 50 ml/100 gm brain tissue/min. However, CBF is not uniform; grey matter has higher values and white matter lower. There are also regional differences related to neuronal activities, both for motor activities and mental endeavors.

The spinal cord is part of the central nervous system, but differs in several ways. First, the total blood flow is usually lower than that in the cerebrum and cerebellum. Second, the spinal cord has the grey matter (with relatively high flow) in the center and is surrounded by white matter; in the cerebrum it is the reverse. Third, the perfusion to the brain is via four large arteries; in the spinal cord several smaller arteries from various levels form the posterior and anterior spinal arteries.

Another factor to consider is the close relationship between cerebral blood flow (CBF) and intracranial pressure (ICP), especially in cases with space-occupying lesions. In patients with potentially high ICP, anesthesia and techniques used in the ICU can be of significant importance. Anything that will increase CBF (hypertension, hypercapnia, pain, stress, hyperthermia) and thereby ICP should be avoided.

Furthermore, normal regulatory mechanisms exist only if homeostasis is maintained. Severe hypoxia, ischemia, trauma, brain tumors, or certain drugs (osmotic drugs, chemotherapy) may alter or abolish normal autoregulation and the function of the blood brain barrier (BBB); these may make perfusion of the central nervous system (CNS) dependent on other factors. If the BBB is disrupted, then drugs and metabolites may enter the brain and cause unexpected or unwanted effects (1-5).

SITUATIONS WITH POTENTIAL RISK
FOR CEREBRAL ISCHEMIA

Diagnostic neuroradiologic procedures are very often overlooked. Patients are sent for tests to obtain anatomical or functional information and the expectation of a complication is very low. To gain the most information, patients may be positioned so that perfusion is hampered by constricted flow. If there is a need for sedation the risk from the unprotected airway--hypoxia or hypercapnia--is added. It is recommended that patients with potentially compromised cerebral circulation should have sufficient monitoring to prevent such incidents.

Another illustrative situation involves acute increases in intracranial pressure (ICP). If blood flow to a cerebral region is at its lower limit, any reduction in the cerebral perfusion pressure (CPP = MABP - ICP) may result in regional ischemia. The anesthesiologist is aware that his induction agent should not lower the blood pressure dramatically. The quoted formula, however, shows that an increase in the ICP will have the same detrimental effect. During anesthesia and surgery there are two particular times when an unwanted increase in ICP could occur. The first is during intubation. It is well documented that intubation is associated with a potential increase in arterial blood pressure (6-9), which will affect both MABP and central venous pressure (and secondarily the ICP). The combined effect may very well be a drop in CPP. The second situation is with surgical start and incision. Again the stimulation changes central pressures, and potentially the CPP. In vascular beds where there are limitations, changes in perfusion pressure can lead to ischemia.

PAIN AND STRESS

The potential effect on the CPP from a sudden increase in blood pressure was mentioned in the previous section. It is not only in the operating room where this can happen. In the intensive care unit (ICU), patients are under stress and even sometimes encounter pain. In animal studies stress and pain have been shown to be associated with increases in cerebral blood flow and cerebral metabolism (10,11). This is most likely due to passage of catecholamines into the brain (4,5). When the metabolic demands are increased, it is important that the supply of oxygen and substrates not be limited, or otherwise an imbalance will occur with ischemic changes as a consequence.

PHYSIOLOGIC PARAMETERS

Regulation of CBF is not yet fully understood, but several factors that influence the flow are known. Most studied and of greatest importance for the anesthesiologist/intensivist are various physiologic parameters, like blood pressure (see above), temperature (12,13), hemoglobin concentration (14,15), oxygen content (16,17), carbon dioxide content and pH (5,18).

In patients with limited circulatory reserve (e.g., stenosis of extracranial or intracranial arteries) a drop in blood pressure, a drop in hemoglobin, or a fall in oxygen concentration are the most detrimental. They all lead to an imbalance between supply and demand.

The most commonly seen change in body temperature in the operating room and in the ICU is a decrease. A drop in temperature will lower CBF. On the other hand, it will also lower the metabolic demand, so this change is less dangerous. Carbon dioxide is a potent vasodilator. Normally a change in $PaCO_2$ of 1 mm Hg will change the blood flow by 5% (5). Effects on abnormal vessels are less well known; in fact, a cerebral steal phenomenon may occur if other areas are more reactive to CO_2 levels.

When PaCO$_2$ is chronically elevated, an adaptation of the CSF level of bicarbonate occurs, with a tendency to normalize pH in spinal fluid, and with that a normalization of tone in the cerebral circulation (19-21). These changes occur over 2-3 days, and any acute changes instituted in hypercapnic patients may lead to acute imbalances in regulatory mechanisms with subnormal levels of CBF for periods of time. In patients with chronically elevated PaCO$_2$ levels, all changes must be done very carefully.

CEREBRAL ISCHEMIA AND CEREBRAL STEAL

Ischemia occurs when blood flow is too low to furnish enough oxygen to support various cellular functions. In humans normal cerebral blood flow averages about 50 ml/100 g tissue/min. During induced hypotension a drop in CBF to about 30 ml/100 g/min induces symptoms such as somnolence, dizziness, and initiation of hyperventilation (22). In lightly anesthetized humans with temporary occlusion of the carotid artery the electroencephalogram (EEG) showed early flattening at CBF levels of 20 ml/100 g/min (23,24). In primates similar studies showed the same findings at CBFs of 18-20 ml/100 g/min (25). There is thus evidence that the ischemic flow for disruption of neuronal transmission is close to 20 ml/100 g/min.

Below this threshold there appears to be another level at about 8-10 ml/100 g/min--the ischemic level of metabolic failure (26,27). Below 10 ml/100 g/min, significant changes occur on levels of intracellular potassium, phosphocreatine and adenosine triphosphate (28-30). If such ischemia is sustained, an ischemic necrosis is very likely. The interesting discussion today is about the "gray zone" between 20 and 10 ml/100 g/min. Astrup et al (26) have given this zone the name **ischemic penumbra**, since it has been shown that some recovery of function occurs even after very prolonged periods of severe depression of CBF (27,31,32). Neurosurgical techniques (e.g., temporary arterial clips or pressure from retractors) may be proof of the same.

Any episode of inadequate perfusion of the brain leads to the rapid production of lactic acidosis followed by a loss of autoregulation of CBF and potentially to a dissociation of blood flow and metabolism. In the ischemic region paradoxical changes in the blood flow can be identified as **steal**, **reverse steal**, or **false autoregulation** (33). Cerebral steal is a condition where vasodilatation in adjacent areas diverts blood from the ischemic areas. This occurs if potent vasodilators, like hypercapnia or papaverine, open up the flow to regions with normal reactivity while the passive region cannot react. The converse occurs if vasoconstriction lowers the flow to the normal region and diverts blood to the ischemic, passive region. Hypocapnia and theophylline infusions can cause reverse steal. False autoregulation is a phenomenon not yet understood. For example, in patients with head injury the area of the contusion has an abolished or a paradoxical reaction to CO_2 while autoregulation to blood pressure changes is maintained.

CLINICAL CORRELATIONS

Even if some of the previously mentioned studies have quoted preserved brain activity after extremely long ischemic periods (27,31,32), intraoperative ischemia must certainly still be avoided. In patients with potential risk for ischemia of the brain, such as patients with carotid stenosis, everything should be done to maintain normal cerebral blood flow during non-neurosurgical procedures.

It is clear from the previous presentation that increased demands on the cerebral circulation should be avoided. Hypoxia, anemia, hyperthermia, hypercapnia, stress and pain all increase CBF. Changes in the other direction are also to be avoided. Hypocapnia or a fall in blood pressure can dramatically limit cerebral blood flow in this group of patients. Thus, induction of anesthesia has to be stable, but must also assure sufficient anesthesia to blunt the blood pressure increase seen with intubation.

Of available induction agents thiopental has the advantage in that it lowers the metabolic demand; the negative effect is that in some patients thiopental can lower the blood pressure, even for prolonged periods of time. Neuroleptanalgesia is a technique where droperidol is given together with fentanyl. This combination is given slowly until the patient becomes unresponsive, at which time the patient can be intubated. The advantage is that high doses of narcotics will blunt the stress response, but disadvantages are that droperidol lowers the blood pressure by vasodilatation and that induction is slow and depresses respiration. An alternative to the second technique is to use the so-called "high dose narcotic" technique, where narcotics are given by infusion in such doses that the patient becomes unresponsive within a few minutes. Cardiovascular stability is usually maintained, but again respiration is impaired, chest wall rigidity can be a problem, and for short cases the postoperative respiratory depression may be a negative factor. Some modern techniques include use of midazolam (a short-acting benzodiazepine) and etomidate (a non-barbiturate sedative/hypnotic). They both provide relatively stable hemodynamics. One side effect of etomidate is a significant depression in cortisol production for at least 24 hours.

Anesthesiologists often combine several drugs and anesthetic gases to achieve pharmacologic effects. Maintenance of anesthesia can be accomplished with either a continuous infusion of some of the previous agents, or with inhalational anesthetics. All available anesthetic gases have a vasodilatory effect on CBF. With limitations in CBF, any change may cause steal or reverse steal, so the recommendation is to use the volatile agent with the least cerebral vasodilatation. Today that is isoflurane.

It is also necessary to monitor and to control physiologic parameters to some degree. Long procedures require measures to keep the patient's body temperature close to normal--a warming blanket, warmed i.v. solutions, and an "artificial nose" or warm air humidifier in the breathing circuit. An arterial catheter allows continuous measurement of the blood pressure, and also makes it possible to obtain arterial blood gases for adjustment of ventilation.

SUMMARY

Patients with restricted blood flow to the brain are at risk for ischemia when under anesthesia and surgery for other procedures. They should be evaluated for this risk prior to surgery, the head should be kept in a neutral position, physiologic parameters should be monitored and adjusted, and anesthetic techniques should be chosen so as to preserve normal blood flow to the brain.

ACKNOWLEDGEMENTS

The writing of this review article was supported in part by Biomedical Research Support Grant SO7 RR05417 from the Division of Research Resources, National Institute of Health. Dr. Wendling is the recipient of an Anesthesiology Young Investigator Award from the Foundation for Anesthesia Education and Research and Janssen Pharmaceutica.

REFERENCES

1.   Steinwall, O., I. Klatzo, Selective vulnerability of the blood-brain barrier in chemically induced lesions. *J. Neuropathol. Exp. Neurol.*, 1966; 25: 542-559

2.   Carlsson, A.:Amphetamine and brain catecholamines. Costa E, Garattini S (eds.): Amphetamines and related compounds. Raven Press, New York, 1970; 289-300

3.   Partridge, W.M.: Brain metabolism: a perspective from the blood-brain barrier. *Physiol. Rev.*, 1983; 63: 1481-1535

4.   MacKenzie, E.T., J. McCulloch, M. O'Keane, J.D. Pichard, A.M. Harper, Cerebral circulation and norepinephrine: relevance of the blood-brain barrier. *Am. J. Physiol.*, 1976; 231: 483-488

5.   MacKenzie, E.T., J. McCulloch, A.M. Harper, Influence of endogenous norepinephrine on cerebral blood flow and metabolism. *Am. J. Physiol.*, 1976; 231: 489-494

6.   Curran, J., M. Crowley, G. O'Sullivan, Droperidol and endotracheal intubation. Attenuation of pressure response to laryngoscopy and intubation. *Anesthesia*, 1980; 35: 290-294

7.   Werner, O., J. Magnusson, R. Fletcher, C. Carlsson, K.I. Pettersson, Effect of cardioselective beta-blockers on the heart rate and arterial pressure response to laryngoscopy. *Acta Anaesthesiol. Scand.*, 1982; 26 (Suppl. 76): 78-80

8.   Chen, C.T., T.J.K. Toung, R.T. Donham, Fentanyl dosage of suppression of circulatory response to laryngoscopy and endotracheal intubation. *Anesth. Rev.*, 1986; 13: 37-42

9.   Liu, P.L., S. Gatt, L.D. Gugino, S.R. Mallampi, B.G. Covino, Esmolol for control of increase in heart rate and blood pressure during tracheal intubation after thiopentone and succinylcholine. *Can. Anaesth. Soc. J.*, 1986; 33: 556-565

10.   Carlsson, C., M. Hagerdal, A.E. Kaasik, B.K. Siesjo, A catecholamine mediated increase in cerebral oxygen uptake during immobilization stress in rats. *Brain Res.*, 1976; 199: 223-231

11.   Bryan, R.M. Jr., R.A. Hawkins, A.M. Mans, D.W. Davis, R.B. Page, Cerebral glucose utilization in awake unstressed rats. *Am. J. Physiol.*, 1983; 244: C270-C275

12.   Hagerdal, M., J.R. Harp, L. Nilsson, B.K. Siesjo, The effect of induced hypothermia upon oxygen consumption in the rat brain. *J. Neurochem.*, 1975; 24: 311-316

13.   Carlsson, C., M. Hagerdal, B.K. Siesjo, The effect of hyperthermia upon oxygen consumption and upon organic phosphates, glycolytic metabolites, citric acid cycle intermediates and associated amino acids in the rat cerebral cortex. *J. Neurochem.*, 1976; 26: 1001-1112

14.   Johannsson, H., B.K. Siesjo, Blood flow and oxygen consumption in the rat brain in dilutional anemia. *Acta Physiol. Scand.*, 1974; 91: 136-138

15.   Johannsson, H., B.K. Siesjo, Brain energy metabolism in anesthetized rats in acute anemia. *Acta Physiol. Scand.*, 1975; 93: 515-525

16.   Eklof, B., N.A. Lassen, L. Nilsson, K. Norberg, B.K. Siesjo, Blood flow and metabolic rate for oxygen in the cerebral cortex of the rat. *Acta Physiol. Scand.*, 1973; 88: 587-589

17.   Dahlgren, N. Local cerebral blood flow in spontaneously breathing rats subjected to graded isobaric hypoxia. *Acta Anaesth. Scand.*, 1990; 34: 463-467

18.   Norberg, K., B.K. Siesjo, Quantitative measurement of blood flow and oxygen consumption in the rat brain. *Acta Physiol. Scand.*, 1974; 91: 154-164

19.   Christensen, M.S., P. Brodersen, J. Olesen, O.B. Poulsen, Cerebral apoplexy (stroke) treated with or without prolonged artificial hyperventilation. II. Cerebrospinal fluid acid-base balance and intracranial pressure. *Stroke*, 1973; 4: 620-631

20.   Fencl, V., J.R. Vale, J.A. Brock, Respiration and cerebral blood flow in metabolic acidosis and alkalosis in humans. *J. Appl. Physiol.*, 1969; 27: 67-76

21.   Pannier, J.L., J. Wayne, G. Demeester, Influence of changes in the acid-base composition of the ventricular system on cerebral blood flow in cats. *Pflugers Arch.*, 1972; 333: 337-351

22. Baron, J.-C., D. Rougemont, M.G. Bousser, Local CBF, oxygen extraction fraction (OEF) and $CMRO_2$: Prognostic value in recent supratentorial infarction in humans. *J. Cereb. Blood Flow Metab.*, 1983; 3 (Suppl. 1): 1-2

23. Trojaborg, W., G. Boysen, Relation between EEG, regional cerebral blood flow and internal carotid artery pressure during carotid endarterectomy. *Electroenceph. Clin. Neurophys.*, 1973; 34: 61-69

24. Vorstrup, S.: Tomographic cerebral blood flow measurements in patients with ischemic cerebrovascular disease and evaluation of the vasodilatory capacity by the acetazolamide test. *Acta Neurol. Scand.*, 1988; 77 (Suppl. 114): 1-48

25. Branston, N.M., L. Symon, H.A. Crockard, E. Pazztor, Relationship between the cortical evoked potential and local cortical blood flow following acute middle cerebral artery occlusion in the baboon. *Exp. Neurol.*, 1974; 45: 195-208

26. Astrup, J., B.K. Siesjo, L. Symon, The state of "penumbra" in the ischemic brain: Viable and lethal thresholds in cerebral ischemia (editorial). *Stroke*, 1981; 12: 723-725

27. Morawetz, R.B., T.H. Jones, R.G. Ojemann, F.W. Marcoux, U. De Girolami, R.M. Crowell, Regional cerebral blood flow during temporary middle cerebral artery occlusion in waking monkeys. *Acta Neurol. Scand.*, 1977; 64 (Suppl.): 114-115

28. Astrup, J., G. Blennow, B. Nilsson, Effects of reduced cerebral blood flow upon EEG pattern, cerebral extracellular potassium and energy metabolism in the rat cortex during bicuculline induced seizures. *Brain Res.*, 1979; 177: 115-126

29. Astrup, J., L. Symon, N.M. Branston, N.A. Lassen, Cortical evoked potential and extracellular K^+ and H^+ at critical levels of brain ischemia. *Stroke*, 1977; 8: 51-57

30. Branston, N.M., A.J. Strong, L. Symon, Extracellular potassium activity, evoked potential and tissue blood flow. *J. Neurol. Sci.*, 1977; 32: 305-321

31. Hossman, V., K.-A. Hossman, Return of neuronal function after prolonged cardiac arrest. *Brain Res.*, 1973; 60: 423-428

32.   Hossman, K.-A., V. Zimmerman, Resuscitation of the monkey brain after 1 hour complete ischemia. I. Physiological and morphological observations. *Brain Res.*, 1974; 81: 59-74

33.   Enevoldsen, E., F.T. Jensen, Autoregulation and CO_2 responses of cerebral blood flow in patients with acute severe head injury. *J. Neurosurg.*, 1978: 48: 689-703

7

CRITICAL CARE MANAGEMENT OF NEUROVASCULAR PROBLEMS: PRACTICAL AND THEORETICAL CONSIDERATIONS

Robert H. Rosenwasser, M.D., F.A.C.S.
Associate Professor of Neurological Surgery
and Physiology
Director, Neurological Intensive Care Unit
Temple University Hospital
Philadelphia, Pa.

INTRODUCTION

This chapter will deal with disease entities whose morbidity is directly related to cerebral ischemia. It will include subarachnoid hemorrhage, head injury, stroke and stroke in evolution, although stroke will be discussed in detail in the following chapter.

SUBARACHNOID HEMORRHAGE

Subarachnoid hemorrhage accounts for approximately 25% of all deaths which involve primary central nervous system events related to intracranial hemorrhage. In North America, intracranial bleeding is responsible for approximately 50% of deaths from stroke. There are 28,000 cases of subarachnoid hemorrhage per year in North America. Approximately 10,000 die from the initial insult and never make it to a hospital. That leaves 18,000 patients available for treatment; however, 3,000 die from the effects of rebleeding and 3,000 die from vasospasm (4-7). An additional 3,000 succumb to medical and surgical complications relative to their subarachnoid hemorrhage.

                        Robert H. Rosenwasser

POST-SURGICAL RESULTS

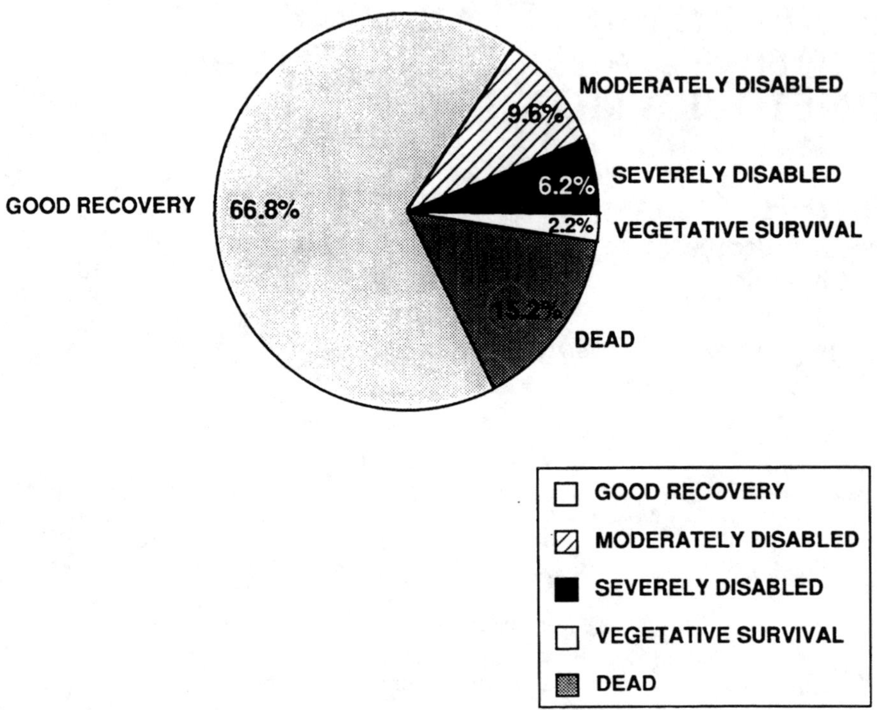

Figure 1A.

That leaves 9,000 patients who leave the hospital and, according to some studies, only 30% of that group return to their premorbid occupation (98,99).

COMPLICATIONS OF SUBARACHNOID HEMORRHAGE

The cooperative aneurysm study was very revealing in its outcome results in the post-surgical group as well as overall results (Figure 1A, 1B) (8,11,98). The outcome was measured according to the Glasgow Outcome Scale, and the post-surgical results demonstrated that good recovery was demonstrated in only 66.8% of the patients, with moderate disability in 9.6%, severe disability in 6.2%, vegetative survival in 2.2%, with a mortality in that group of 15.2%. Overall results at three months demonstrated good recovery of 56.4%, moderate disability of 8.4%, severe disability of 5.7%, vegetative survival in 2.2% and an overall mortality of 27.3%. This data must be looked at very carefully, in that management of patients with subarachnoid hemorrhage has evolved dramatically over the past decade since these statistics were gathered and published. Patients are now routinely managed with calcium channel blockers, primarily Nimodipine which will be discussed later, as well as hypervolemic hemodilution which is a mainstay of therapy concerning fluid management (8,11,98). The decision regarding early or late surgery is still controversial, although many centers are leaning toward early operation, defined as within the first 48 hours after the initial ictus (164,208,209).

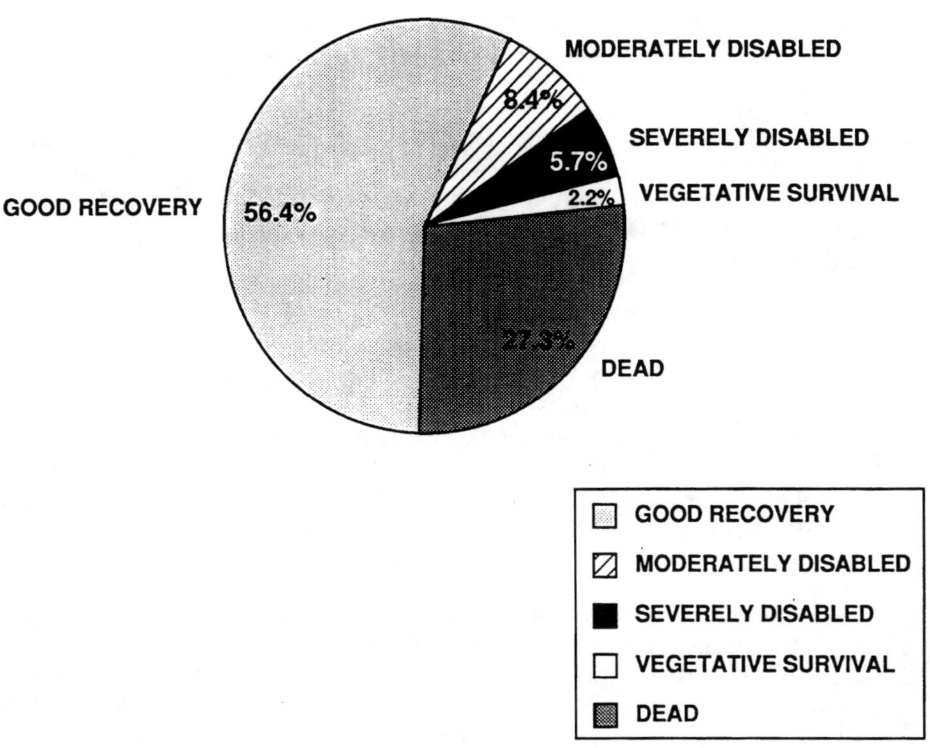

Figure 1B.

The complications of subarachnoid hemorrhage are generally divided into the management of elevated intracranial pressure (132-134), arterial hypertension, re-hemorrhage from an unsecured aneurysm, and cerebral vasospasm. The management of these complications must be undertaken with an understanding of the pathophysiology of cerebral ischemia and reperfusion in mind. In a patient with either elevated intracranial hypertension and/or cerebral vasospasm, what one is trying to preserve is the ischemic penumbra (132,133). The goal is to provide a therapeutic intervention to restore cerebral blood flow and membrane homeostasis. In the patient with either long-standing intracranial hypertension and/or vasospasm, one must consider the no reflow phenomenon, where swelling of perivascular glial cells occurs as well as swelling of endothelial tissue with bleb formation and compression of capillaries, further causing stagnant blood with resultant ischemia (37). There is the question of increased viscosity at the capillary level, and there is data to suggest that the no reflow may be attenuated with hemodilution (137,150). In addition, the concept of delayed hyperperfusion should be considered. There are intravascular factors which may occur due to endothelial swelling and endothelial blood interactions, and these may be manipulated by rheologic means (59), which will be discussed. There are significant structural and biochemical changes in the endothelium with reduction of prostacyclin, which may potentiate vessel constriction and platelet activation, further impeding the flow of blood to the cellular structures (12,20,84,97,104,105).

INCREASED INTRACRANIAL PRESSURE

Thoughts concerning the role of intracranial pressure survival following head injury go back hundreds of years. Monro, in the late 1700's, published a treatise in which he attempted to establish the relationship between pressure and volume within the closed cranial cavity (131). His original thesis concerned brain and blood within the closed cranial cavity but he did not consider the cerebrospinal fluid, and Kellie later expounded on Monro's original thoughts (103). However, it was Burrows in the 1840's who considered cerebrospinal fluid, blood and brain tissue all important in the pressure volume relationship (34). The Monro-Kellie doctrine essentially states that volume is constant in the closed cranial cavity and that any change in one of the compartments must cause a compensatory reciprocal change in the other two. Mathematically this is defined as $Vc = X + Y + Z + Zi$; x is brain tissue, y is blood volume and z is cerebro-spinal fluid , and Zi is any other intracranial space occupying mass such as a subdural/extradural or intracerebral hematoma.

The total intracranial volume in adults is approximately 2000 cc's, 80% being parenchymal tissue, 10% blood volume and 10% cerebral spinal fluid. It is the surgical manipulation of brain tissue and the pharmacological and physiological manipulation of blood volume and cerebrospinal fluid that are key in the ability to control non-physiological levels of intracranial pressure.

Although methods of measuring intracranial pressure were explored in the 1930's, it was not until 1960 when Lundberg published his classic work on continuous ventricular monitoring that normal values of intracranial pressure wave forms were categorized (118). These have been termed "Lundberg Waves" and have been classified as A (percussion wave), B (tidal wave), and C (dichrotic waves). A waves or plateau waves are pathological, reflecting severe pathological elevation of intracranial pressure that begins from a normal base line and may increase to 50 mm Hg and last anywhere from three to thirty minutes, usually terminating with an abrupt return to baseline. Unless the pathological process causing the elevated pressure is corrected, these plateau waves will be repetitive causing multiple small infarcts as a result of repetitive episodes of ischemia.

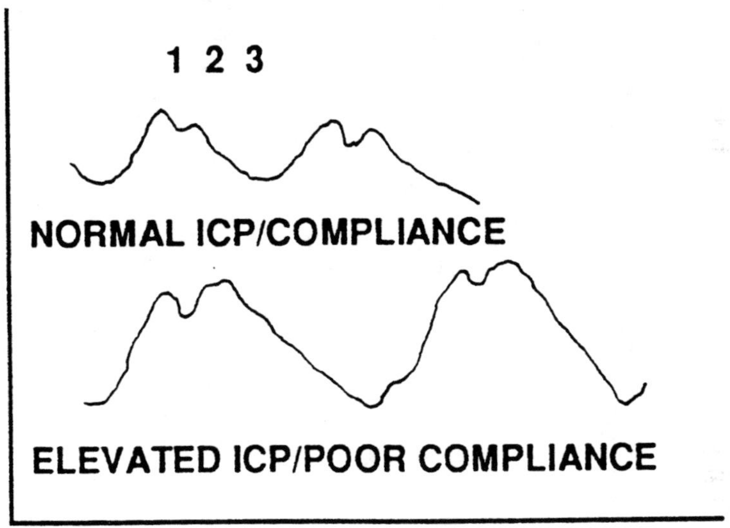

Figure 2.

B waves generally occur at one to two per minute with amplitude being greater than 10-20 mm Hg. B waves reflect the influence of respiration on ICP and also indicate a moderately compromised intracranial reserve and reduced compliance. They do not carry the serious prognosis of A waves; however they are significant as warning signs for marked reduction in compliance and may signify impending A waves.

C waves show a slow oscillation in blood pressure and are repetitive over the respiratory cycle.   In general they reflect arterial curves of Traube-Hering (refer to Figure 2).

Miller *et. al.* (129) and Monro *et. al.* (131) had provided valuable information for quantification of pressure volume relationships as they relate to control and management of intracranial pressure.   These authors have evolved the concept of intracranial compliance and the pressure volume index (PVI) (Figure 3).   The PVI defines the change in intracranial pressure resulting from increase or decrease in small volumes of intraventricular fluid and is directly proportional to the amount of compliance in the intracranial compartment.   This relationship is defined as

$$PVI = \frac{V}{\log Po/P}$$

where V is volume of fluid added or withdrawn, Po is the baseline ICP prior to manipulation and P delta is the ICP following manipulation.   Maset et al reported that patients with values of 20 ml or greater require only minimal ICP therapy, whereas patients whose PVI ranges from 15-20 ml are prone to have significant elevations of intracranial pressure, and patients with PVI values less than 15 ml require intensive ICP therapy and are at highest risk for developing intractable ICP (125).

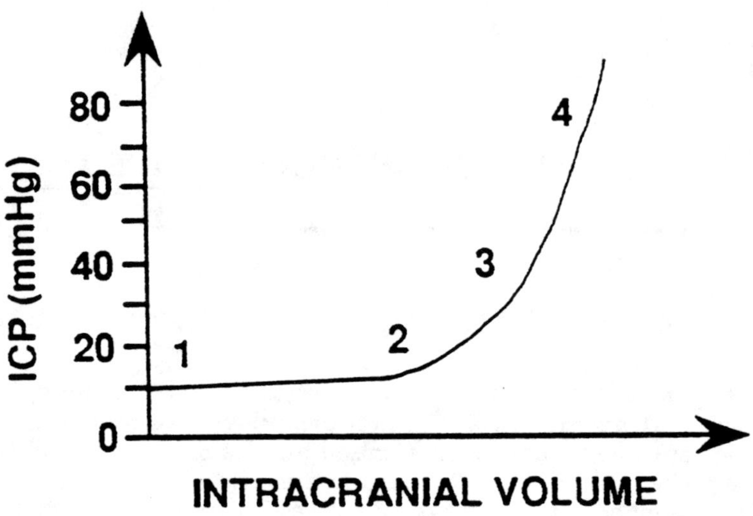

Figure 3A.

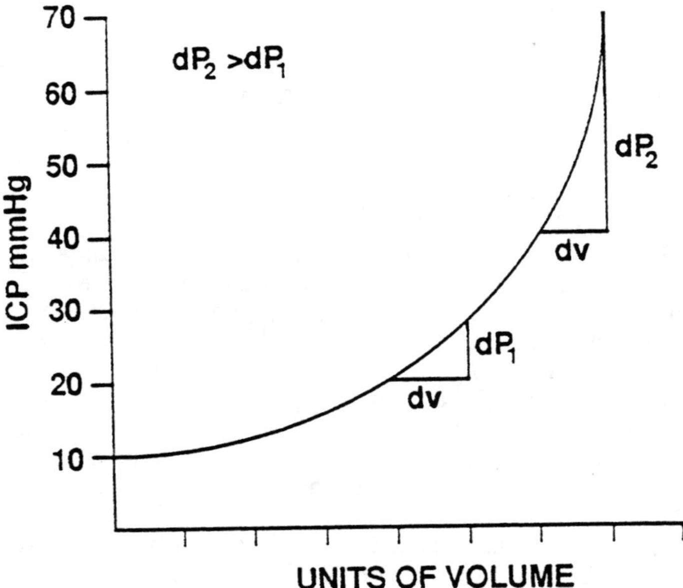

Figure 3B.

THE ROLE OF INTRACRANIAL PRESSURE MONITORING

Controversy abounds concerning the role of intracranial pressure monitoring, and whether it alters outcome. It is known that approximately 40% of patients with loss of consciousness due to head injury develop intracranial hypertension (159,236).   Fifty percent of multiple trauma patients who die do so from intractable intracranial hypertension. According to the National Traumatic Coma Data Bank, ICP was a predictor of outcome according to the Glasgow outcome score. It appeared to be statistically independent of other predicted factors such as admission motor score, age, and pupillary exam. Rosner *et. al.* (173) and Tsutsume *et. al.* (227) have argued that cerebral perfusion pressure (CPP) should be the actual parameter of interest in the head injured patient and, in fact, that CPP should replace ICP. However, Marmarou et al performed multiple regression analysis of data from the National Traumatic Coma Data Bank and found ICP to be predictive of outcome, independent of cerebral perfusion (120,235). Despite the controversy, there is evidence that, in the population of patients with moderate to severe head injury, treatment of intracranial hypertension is associated with improved outcome at six months. Narayan et al demonstrated that expected treatment of small incremental rises in ICP perhaps prevents development of unacceptable levels of ICP (140). Marshall et al presented similar data that outcome is improved with patients whose ICP was maintained below 15 millimeters of mercury as compared to those whose ICP exceeded 40 millimeters of mercury for greater than or equal to fifteen minutes (122,123). Saul and Ducker demonstrated improved outcome for patients treated at an ICP of 15 compared to 25 mm Hg (181). The role of ICP in head injury must be discussed concomitantly with the regulation of the cerebral circulation and its metabolism. It is well known that normal CBF is approximately 50cc/100 gm/minute. The O_2 content of arterial blood is approximately 14 cc per deciliter of arterial blood. The arterial-venous difference of oxygen (A-VO_2) is 6.3 cc per deciliter. Knowing the cerebral blood flow and the AV oxygen difference, one can calculate the metabolic rate of oxygen consumption of the brain otherwise termed CMR 02 (CMR 02 = CBF x A-V02). Two mechanisms exist in which the brain attempts to maintain homeostasis and prevent energy failure. The first is to increase the arteriovenous oxygen difference when flow decreases. Compensation for oxygen extraction can occur at a flow of approximately 23 cc/100 gm/minute. Below this flow, energy failure occurs with associated neuronal and glial dysfunction and resultant cell death. The second mechanism involves oxygen extraction at a constant level but maintenance of cerebral blood flow despite reduction in perfusion pressure from either low arterial pressure or elevated intracranial pressure. This is referred to as metabolic autoregulation. References on cerebral autoregulation are included for the interested reader (2,45,186,202,211,212,214,217,220,239).

Cerebral blood flow is expressed according to the Poiseuille equation

$$CBF = K \times \frac{(\text{mean arterial BP} - ICP)D4}{8 \ VL}$$

where K is a constant and the length of the blood vessel L does not change. Cerebral blood flow is essentially determined by changes in the mean arterial blood pressure (MABP), ICP, blood viscosity, and the diameter of the arteries and arterioles (D). It is important to understand cerebral blood flow only as it relates to the cerebral perfusion pressure (CPP). The CPP defines the difference between the mean arterial pressure and the intracranial pressure; i.e. CPP is equal to MAP-ICP. Increasing ICP therefore may be responsible for extension of secondary ischemic injury that occurs with intracranial hypertension. It is important to maintain systemic arterial blood pressure to provide a CPP of approximately 70 to 110 mm Hg to insure adequate blood flow to the brain and maximize oxygen substrate.

MANAGEMENT OF INCREASED
INTRACRANIAL PRESSURE

The treatment of elevated intracranial pressure involves modalities of patient position, the respiratory system and pharmacological manipulation as well (47,120,133,135,136, 230,241,243,245). The use of sedation and paralysis, hyperventilation, cerebral spinal fluid drainage, osmotic therapy, diuretics, steroids and barbiturates will be discussed.

HEAD ELEVATION

One of the simple measures that can be employed to treat ICP is head elevation to approximately 30 to 45 degrees. In general, ideal head position can be determined for each patient with the simple maneuver of raising and lowering the bed and observing ICP. In patients who are obese, an extremely elevated position will cause increased abdominal pressure with inferior vena caval compression, resulting in increased intrathoracic pressure and restriction of venous return. Extreme head turning should be avoided, so as not to kink the internal jugular venous system. Great care should be taken in observing the blood pressure during trials of head elevation.

SEDATION AND PARALYSIS

It is a well known phenomenon that pain and agitation exacerbate intracranial hypertension (112,138,225,235,245). Therefore judicious use of analgesics and sedatives is highly recommended as a cornerstone in the control of intracranial pressure. The neurological exam is often obscured by sedatives; however, in the face of elevated intracranial pressure, other modalities of following the neurological status are available such as evoked responses, which will be discussed in a later section. It is unwise to paralyze the patient without the concomitant use of sedation.

Gagging on the endotracheal tube or "bucking" the ventilator is extremely worrisome and can cause an extreme rise in intrathoracic pressure followed by a rise in ICP. The sedation used in our unit consists of Pavulon 4 mg IV p.r.n. every 2-4 hours, followed with Morphine sulfate, 1-5 mg p.r.n. The advantage of narcotic sedation is that it can easily be reversed to clinically assess the neurological status. In addition, prior to suctioning, the level of sedation should be assessed; this can easily be done by gently moving the endotracheal tube. If the pulse increases noticeably or the ICP elevates, the patient should have additional sedation and paralyzation prior to suctioning. The usual dose of 50-100mg of Lidocaine as an aerosol down the endotracheal tube may also may be beneficial in blocking this PCO2 reflex.

Manipulation of the PCO2 by hyperventilation can be accomplished to induce hypocapnia and has been shown to be an effective method of reducing cerebral edema when post-traumatic vasoparalysis has resulted in an increase in cerebral blood volume. Hyperventilation can either be done mechanically by increasing the volume setting of the ventilator or by rapidly ventilating the patient manually with an ambu bag. It is generally accepted that a PCO2 level between 25-30 mm Hg is a potent vasoconstrictor that dramatically reduces the intracranial pressure by reducing the cerebral blood volume due to vasoconstriction. It has been demonstrated that there is no additional benefit in hyperventilating to less than a PCO2 of 25 mm Hg. One wishes to avoid severe vasoconstriction which may result in cerebral ischemia. In addition it has been suggested that the effect of hyperventilation may wear off with time due to buffering of CSF pH, and therefore, if ICP can be controlled with other measures, a slow wean toward normocapnia should be attempted, such that if spikes of ICP recur it can be used again as an acute tool to reduce such pressure elevations (138). In addition, abrupt cessation of hyperventilation may result in rebound vasodilatation and deleterious rises in ICP. In a standard fashion, mechanical ventilation should be managed with paralyzation and sedation and in doses of Pancuronium Bromide 2-4 mg IV every 1-2 hours as necessary and should be accompanied in general by narcotic analgesia and sedation. Volume cycle ventilators are ideal for the management of elevated intracranial pressure, but there are certain occasions where high frequency jet ventilation (HFJV) may be a preferred mode of ventilation (33,40-42,183). There has been no absolute scientific data that HFJV is superior to standard measures of controlled ventilation where elevated ICP is concerned. In patients who require extremely high values of positive end expiratory pressures for adequate oxygenation, HFJV may play a role. This will be discussed further under the section of respiratory complications.

CSF DRAINAGE

There are various modalities to monitor intracranial pressure such as a ventricular catheter, subarachnoid bolt or fiberoptic device (206,225). However in our unit, the ventricular catheter is the device of choice, as it is both therapeutic in the ability to withdraw spinal fluid to lower ICP and diagnostic in following the intracranial pressure. The subarachnoid bolt and fiberoptic device, diagnostic tools alone, have disadvantages in terms of occlusion, swollen brain tissue in terms of the bolt, or fiber breakage in other fiberoptic devices. Withdrawal of 0.5 to 2.0 ml of spinal fluid from a non-compliant ventricular system can often have a dramatic effect on lowering the intracranial pressure. If the ventricles become slit-like and occlude the ventricular catheter, it becomes difficult to withdraw fluid. In addition, the wave form may be dampened, in which case a subarachnoid bolt or fiberoptic device may then be placed. In general, ventricular drainage should be instituted concomitantly with the use of hyperventilation and/or osmotic therapy (47,141,157,166,169,236,237).

In our unit, we use an entirely closed system and do not access in the ventricular port for fluid sampling. We do, however, sample CSF from the distal portion of the system and perform daily fluid sampling to monitor the CSF white blood cell count. It has been demonstrated that this is the most sensitive indicator of early ventricular infection (126,206). In addition, in our closed system we add 4 mg of intrathecal Gentamycin to the flush solution and this system is treated in a fashion identical to that used for hyperalimentation. All ventriculostomies should be tunneled subcutaneously for a distance of at least 3-4 cm from the burrhole, as it has been shown that this technique also reduces the incidence of infection.

OSMOTIC THERAPY

In our institution, if hyperventilation and CSF drainage are ineffective in lowering the intracranial pressure, we then use a combination of mannitol and furosemide. Wilkinson and co-workers have shown that the ICP lowering effect of combination therapy is synergistic (237).

Osmotic diuretics appear to have more than one mechanism of action. They establish a blood brain osmotic ingredient and reduce extra cellular fluid volume primarily in normal parenchyma, although some literature indicates that these work in damaged tissue as well (22,141). Blood viscosity is reduced with the use of osmotic agents and there is an increase in micro-circulatory flow. In addition, investigators have demonstrated that a reflex vasoconstriction occurs with the administration of mannitol, which in itself lowers the intracranial pressure by reducing blood volume. Mannitol is the osmotic diuretic of choice and is generally given in doses of .25 to 1.0 gm/Kg by bolus injection or constant infusion. It has been shown that a lower dose of .25 gm/Kg is equally effective in lowering the intracranial pressure as larger doses and this small dose may also result in less disturbance of fluid electrolytes and serum osmolality (156). The serum osmolality should be monitored at least every twelve hours and should not be allowed to rise over 310 to 320 milli-osmolar.

Furosemide is the loop diuretic of choice which has been used to manage intracranial pressure (220,237). There is controversy about the dose which is effective; however, a dose of .5 to 1 mg/Kg as an IV bolus can be repeated every six to twelve hours. Osmolality and electrolyte abnormalities are less severe than with mannitol alone. However, potassium homeostasis must be closely followed.

STEROIDS

In the past, steroids such as Dexamethasone have been administered in large doses to patients with head injuries and ICP (43,46,72,75,121,154,182). Numerous studies are now in the literature which fail to support the hypothesis that they improve intracranial hypertension and promote favorable outcomes from brain injury (43,46,182). Therefore, because of complications associated the use of high dose steroids such as immuno-suppression, hypoglycemia and hyperglycemia as well as metabolism, it is recommended that their administration in the setting of head injury be avoided.

BARBITURATE THERAPY

Controversy concerning the use of barbiturate therapy in the treatment of ICP is abounding (52,170,228,234,238). There have been several non-randomized series which demonstrated that high dose barbiturate therapy administered to patients who failed conventional control of intracranial pressure have benefited from its use and have demonstrated improved outcome (14,238). There have been two randomized studies which have demonstrated that when barbiturates are administered prophylactically to patients presumed at high risk for intractable intracranial hypertension there has been no effect. There is also a great deal of controversy at which level barbiturate therapy should be instituted. Several investigators have taken a very aggressive stand and begin barbiturate therapy early; i.e. when the intracranial pressure is 15 mm Hg, the Glasgow Coma score is 8 or less on admission, and admission CT scan shows obliteration of cisterns.

Barbiturate therapy is not without its own risk. Arterial hypotension, myocardial depression, which is of concern in patients who have had myocardial contusions, hypothermia and reduced resistance to infection have all been presumed to be exacerbated by the use of barbiturates. These complications may overshadow the benefit of barbiturate therapy in the control of ICP, unless great care is taken to achieve homeostasis in other organ systems.

Despite complications associated with the use barbiturates, we have recommended that barbiturate therapy be instituted in the patient population at high risk to develop elevated intracranial pressure. This is in a group of patients who have an admission Glasgow Coma score of 8 or less and have obliteration of the subarachnoid cisterns on the admission CT scan, with or without the presence of a surgical intracranial lesion. It is essential that the patient have a normal circulating blood volume prior to the institution of such therapy. A pulmonary artery catheter should be inserted and cardiac index and output should be calculated every 4-6 hours. Systemic vascular resistance should also be followed as this is lowered dramatically by the use of systemic barbiturates. As the barbiturates are administered, intravascular volume should be repleted with an isotonic or hypertonic solution to achieve a euvolemic state.

A loading dose of 5-10 mg/Kg intravenously is administered over 30 minutes. This is generally followed by a constant infusion of 5 mg/Kg per hour. Blood levels are not followed, therefore the patient should have bipolar EEG monitoring to adjust the dose to achieve burst suppression on the electroencephalogram. Approximately six bursts per minute interspersed with electrocerebral silence is indicative of the maximal depression of brain metabolism that can be achieved.

If cardiac depression or mild hypotension ensues, Dobutamine and/or Dopamine may be used to correct the low systemic vascular resistance if intravascular volume is found to be appropriate. If these agents fail, alpha stimulation with levarteranol or phenylephrine may be employed.

ADDITIONAL PHARMACOLOGICAL AGENTS

LIDOCAINE

Lidocaine has been shown to decrease the rate of synaptic transmission presumably by blockade of sodium channels. In addition, it may have a vasoconstrictor effect as well. It has been shown to decrease cerebral glucose consumption as well as the metabolic rate of oxygen consumption, and has been used in neuroanesthesia to lower ICP associated with intubation and surgical manipulation (17,49,55). Most of these studies have been experimental and its value in the treatment of humans is controversial. As previously mentioned, Lidocaine does diminish acute elevations of ICP associated with nasogastric and nasotracheal suctioning, and as previously outlined, should be administered prophylactically before such bedside procedures are performed.

INVESTIGATIONAL AGENTS

Excitatory Amino Acids

Excitatory amino acids have been implicated in the pathogenesis of injury associated with traumatic and ischemic brain conditions (23,149). Glutamate is a known excitatory amino acid with wide distributions and high concentrations in brain tissue (100,101,139,144). It is known that glutamate agonists potentiate ischemic injury. There are three types of glutamate receptors which are the N-methyl D-aspartate (NMDA), quisqualate and the kainate receptors. Up to an eight-fold increase in extracellular glutamate has been measured in ischemic rat hippocampus. The development of agents that can block glutamate receptor mediated injury are underway (160). These are primarily involving the NMDA receptor which block calcium influx which is known to cause an active cascade of ischemic injury (57). Currently, NMDA receptor antagonists are being studied in clinical trials, but at this time cannot be recommended for general use (13).

Lactate

It is known that ischemia and hypoxia secondary to traumatic lesions and subarachnoid hemorrhage lead to marked derangements of energy metabolism with resultant acidosis (106). There have been many studies which have monitored cerebrospinal fluid and cerebral venous lactate (106,201,216). It has been found to be elevated in numerous animal and human studies where head injury was present. The lactate concentration has been found to be proportional to the severity of injury in humans, and in some studies has been used as a predictor of outcome. Several drugs have been administered systemically, and one of the most promising appears to be trishydroxymethyl aminomethane (THAM). This agent is a systemic and intracellular alkalinizing agent that has been studied in animal models and in humans with head injury. Several of these studies have demonstrated a marked lowering of intracranial pressure with resultant decreased morbidity and improved survival. A randomized study using THAM is currently under way (172,174).

Free Radicals

Free radicals are a species of compounds that are known to have a free electron in the outer shell and are formed during normal anaerobic metabolism (29,60,187). When metabolic homeostasis is present, these stray electrons are neutralized by naturally occurring antioxidants. In the face of ischemia, these free electrons can be very deleterious, initiating a sequence of lipid peroxidation with resultant membrane damage and cell death (77). Several agents are under investigation which are presumed free radical scavengers. In particular, there are a group of synthetic 21-amino steroid compounds which lack glucocorticoid activity and appear to be the most promising agent within this novel class of free radical scavengers. This class of free radical scavengers are referred as to lazaroids, and the most promising agent appears to be U-74006F (78-80). Animal studies using this agent have been performed in subarachnoid hemorrhage, cerebral and spinal cord ischemia, spinal cord injury and head injury, all with promising results (78-80,213,244). A multi-center trial using this agent in moderate and severe head injury is currently under way to study its effects on ICP.

VASOSPASM

C. Miller, Fisher et al in 1980 demonstrated that there was a significant correlation between the amount of blood on the CT scan and the development of the clinical syndrome of cerebral vasospasm (61). There was a 99% incidence of severe spasm in patients who had subarachnoid hematomas larger than 5X3 mm, or layers of blood 1 mm or more in any of the cisterns. The pathology of vasospasm has indicated that the arterioles and large conducting arteries show subintimal thickening after prolonged spasm. There is also focal infarction in the territory supplied by the vessel. Interestingly, there is a poor correlation between angiographic cerebral vasospasm and clinical vasospasm. This is related to the fact that cerebral function remains intact until cerebral blood flow falls to 18-20 cc/ 100 grams/minute. In addition, in severe diffuse spasm, there is decreased cerebral blood flow and the $CMRO_2$ is more reduced than the regional cerebral blood flow. It appears that there is an uncoupling between flow and metabolism. Grubb et al have demonstrated that there is an increase in cerebral blood volume with a questionable constriction of large vessels with a dilatation of intraparenchymal vessels (36,74).

MANAGEMENT OF CEREBRAL VASOSPASM

The cornerstone of the treatment of cerebral vasospasm still revolves around intravascular volume augmentation associated with rheologic manipulation of the blood components. Maroon and Nelson, in 1979, documented that there was decreased red cell mass and/or plasma volume in patients with subarachnoid hemorrhage. It was after this point in time that observations were made that suggested that cardiac function, perfusion pressure and blood rheology could perhaps be manipulated with beneficial effects on the ischemic neurologic component of the syndrome referred to as clinical vasospasm. The concept of intravascular fluid manipulation is based on a concept of the Hagen-Poiseuille equation below:

$$Q = \frac{P \; \pi \; R4}{8 \; Ln}$$

where Q is equal to blood, P is the pressure gradient and r is the vessel radius, l is the vessel length and n is the viscosity. The ultimate goal in the patient with clinical vasospasm is to increase the cerebral blood flow by increasing the pressure gradient and/or reducing the blood viscosity, thereby dramatically increasing cerebral blood flow. The factors determining blood viscosity have been defined as the hematocrit, erythrocyte aggregation, erythrocyte flexibility , platelet aggregation, and plasma viscosity. Two of these components which can be manipulated easily are the hematocrit and the plasma viscosity. The act of hemodilution is carried out concurrently, as intravascular volume is expanded. It has been demonstrated that the ideal hematocrit is approximately 30-35 per cent. One can see, from Figure 4, that the ideal hematocrit is approximately 30, at which time the viscosity is minimal and the oxygen transport capacity is the greatest. In normal individuals, cerebral blood flow is determined primarily by the pressure gradient and the radius of the conductance vessels. The same holds true in patients with subarachnoid hemorrhage and one can see that during active episodes of vasospasm the radius is affected dramatically, thereby reducing the flow. If the patient has not yet been operated on for securing of the aneurysm, then increasing blood flow would be safer if done via decreasing viscosity rather than increasing the pressure gradient. In the postoperative period, after the aneurysm has been secured, treatment of spasm can include manipulation of both of these factors.

Kassell et al in described their preliminary results with volume expansion once deficits had become pronounced (179); however, they had a significant rate of complications in 58 patients, with a 17% incidence of pulmonary edema and 19% incidence of aneurysmal rebleeding, and other complications listed in Table X. In this study, the causes of failure were listed as pre-existing infarction in 17%, progression of the vasospasm in 5%, rebleeding in 2% and inability to produce hypertension in 2%.

                    Robert H. Rosenwasser

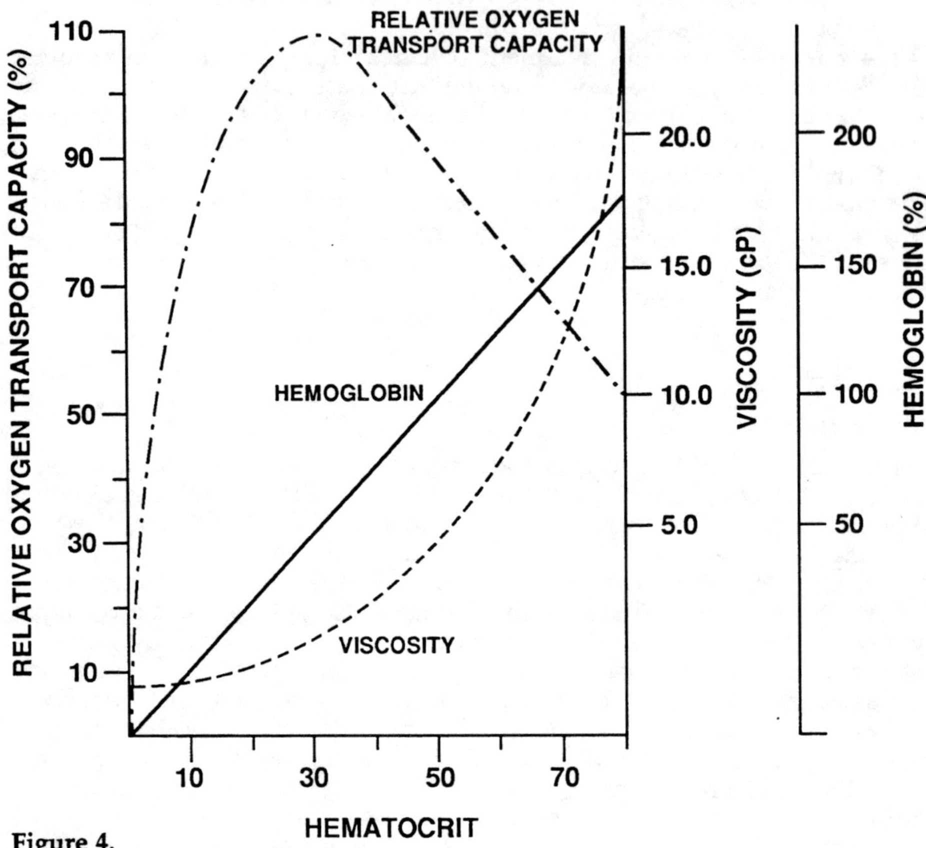

Figure 4.

The problems with acute volume loading became obvious and prophylactic volume expansion was described by Rosenwasser et al in 1983 (168), where Starling curves were calculated for each patient and intravascular volume was increased as blood pressure was concomitantly lowered (Figure 5). Each patient had Starling curves performed routinely every six hours, to determine their own ideal cardiac filling pressures and thereby avoid further complications, such as pulmonary edema. In addition, definitive surgical treatment is generally performed within the first 48 hours, thereby virtually eliminating rebleeding during the treatment of vasospasm (164,208). Table 1 demonstrates the dramatic changes in cerebral blood flow that can be achieved with prophylactic volume expansion and hemodilution.

The diluent of choice is very controversial (167). The debate over colloid and crystalloid continues; however, if one compares cost, crystalloid becomes particularly attractive, as chronic administration of colloid can be extremely expensive. The use of Dextran and hydroxyethyl starch is to be discouraged, in that theseagents, used in large doses, can dramatically affect the coagulation profile and are not approved to be given in a chronic fashion over a 14 day period. Hypertonic saline has some theoretical advantages, in that it reduces endothelial swelling, decreased interstitial water content, readily traverses membrane, thereby avoiding trapping within the pulmonary matrix, improved rheology, and finally is extremely cost effective (177,184,185,193,194,196,205,207). Further studies will be necessary to document effectiveness and safety.

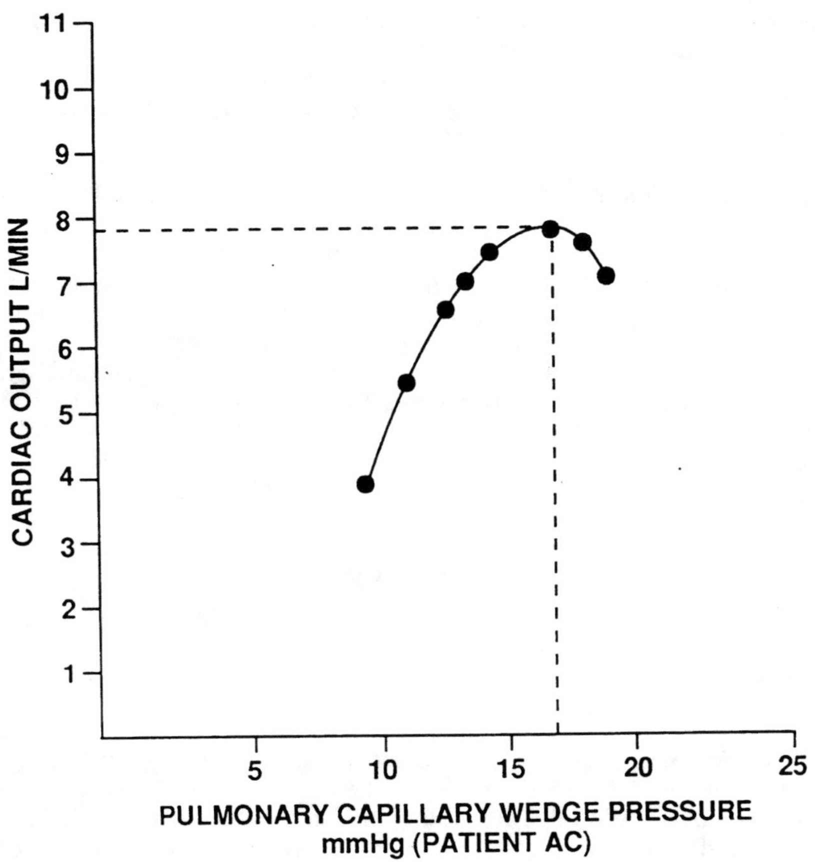

Figure 5.

CALCIUM CHANNEL BLOCKERS

The calcium calmodulin complex has a primary function as it relates to activation of phosphatidylinositol phosphodiesterase which breaks the envelop surrounding a neurotransmitter. In addition, the increased calcium activates phosphorylase a-2 with a ten-fold increase in cytosolic fatty acids (85,86,88,158). With depleted energy stores, such as occurs in cerebral ischemia related to vasospasm, transport of calcium occurs across leaking mitochondrial membranes (178). The process continues until calcium is sequestered in the mitochondria and endoplasmic reticulum. The excess in calcium eventually leads to cell death as the result of membrane disruption. Nimodipine, a 1-4 dihydropyridine derivative, is currently the only approved calcium channel blocker used in North America (18,19,27,67,73,108,240). The dose is 60 mg every four to six hours, and it is given orally. A second drug, Nicardipine, which is an analog, can be given parenterally (62,114,124,151,161,226). These drugs were initially given with the idea that calcium was intricate in smooth muscle relaxation and contraction. With chronic constriction, as seen in cerebral vasospasm, it was initially believed that these drugs would prevent the chronic constriction (221). Although these calcium channel blockers played no role in changing the angiographic appearance of vasospastic vessels (53), in patients who received these agents there was clearly a beneficial effect on morbidity and mortality (26). This was most likely related to the presumed cerebral protective effect of these agents (18,54,233,240). Care must be taken when administering calcium channel antagonists, as one of the major side effects is hypotension (28) and the patients do exhibit a relative hypovolemia which can easily be corrected by intravascular fluid administration.

ARTERIAL HYPERTENSION

With the advent and approval of calcium channel blockers in subarachnoid hemorrhage, they have also been the mainstay of the treatment of hypertension at our institution. Nimodipine doses may be increased accordingly, to maintain a systolic blood pressure of less than or equal to 160 mm Hg. If refractory to these agents, either sodium nitroprusside or trimethaphan, can be administered parenterally in appropriate doses. We have not found this to be necessary, and have been quite satisfied in treating severe hypertension with incremental doses of Nimodipine.

SURVEILLANCE FOR CLINICAL VASOSPASM

The diagnosis of clinical episodes of vasospasm is a diagnosis of exclusion. If the patient is not treated with early operation, re-hemorrhage must be taken into account and a CT scan obtained emergently. In the postoperative period, postoperative hematomas are also a possible cause of clinical deterioration. However, with the advent of transcranial doppler, cerebral blood flow velocities can be monitored, and a rise in the velocity often signifies impending episodes of vasospasm (1,3,66,81,82,87,115,142, 143,162,163,188,189,226,232). Two hundred meters per second is generally considered ultrasonographic evidence of vasospasm; however, the patient should serve as their own control. In general, increase over the patient's velocity by 50-100% in our intensive care unit is taken as active vasospastic episodes. As such, a vigilance is kept at the patient's bedside and great care is taken to avoid hypovolemia, a reduction in the cardiac index and cardiac filling pressures, and treat intracranial hypertension aggressively. It is beyond the scope of this text to discuss the theoretical aspects of transcranial ultrasonography; however, the interested reader is referred to additional references.

There have been various studies that demonstrated that catecholamines are elevated during and after subarachnoid hemorrhage and in periods when the patient has clinical episodes of vasospasm. At our institution, we have studied 300 patients. Two hundred of these were pre-Nimodipine era, 150 of whom were hypertensive and 50 normotensive. We noted that there was an increase in systemic vascular resistance (SVP) in patients who were in clinical vasospasm (165). SVR is defined as

$$\text{(dyne-seconds per cm5)} = \frac{79.96 \times \text{(mean arterial blood pressure - CVP)}}{\text{cardiac output}}$$

In normal individuals, this ranges from 770 to 1500 dyne centimeters per second/cm^5. The results of this study indicated that 42 out of 150 patients, or 28%, developed clinical signs of spasm when they were treated with prophylactic hemodilution and hypervolemia. All patients initially had a high normal PVR and SVR, and that the pulmonary vascular resistance and systemic vascular resistance increased in all patients in clinical spasm. In 38 of the 42 patients, or 90%, the SVR remained elevated as long as clinical signs of spasm persisted. Five out of 50, or 10%, of the normotensive group developed clinical signs of spasm when treated with hypervolemia and hemodilution in a prophylactic fashion. Thirty five of these patients had a high normal SVR and PVR, and when the SVR and PVP returned to normal it was also noted that clinical signs of spasm had abated. This correlated with reduction in transcranial doppler velocities.

The PVR increased in 36 out of 42 patients, or 85%, and remained elevated in 25 of the 42, or 60%. There was no correlation, however, between elevated SVR and PVR and angiographic vasospasm. There was, however, a statistically significant correlation between elevated SVR/PVR and clinical episodes of vasospasm.

COMPLICATIONS OF HEMODYNAMIC MONITORING IN SAH PATIENTS

The critical care literature indicates that the incidence of arterial puncture or hematoma from central venous catheterization is approximately 8%. The incidence of pneumothorax is 2-4%, and hydrothorax 2%. Serious complications such as hemothorax, brachial plexus injury, air embolus, phrenic and recurrent laryngeal nerve damage, and sheared catheter, should collectively be less than 1% incidence (25,39,63,71,89,119,192,199,204). The majority of complications are often related to passage of the catheter. Arrhythmias have been reported to occur anywhere to 13-70%; however, there is only a 1% incidence of serious life-threatening arrhythmias, usually ventricular tachycardia (200). Right bundle branch block has been reported to occur in less than 3% of patients, and cardiac perforation and tamponade less than 1% of the time. When reviewing complications related to an already in-dwelling catheter, infection and/or colonization may occur anywhere from 3-40% of the time, with significant sepsis occurring 4-6% of the time. Thrombosis, with evidence of clinical thromboembolism, generally occurs less than 1% of the time, although there is a 66% incidence of subclavian vein thrombosis. In some series, endocardial damage has been as high as 36%, with valvular damage being less than 1%. Aseptic endocarditis has been reported to occur in upwards of 20% of cases, with bacterial endocarditis being 0-7%. The incidence of pulmonary infarction should also be quite low, with an incidence of 1-7%. Again, pulmonary artery puncture and/or balloon rupture or knotting generally occurs less than 1% of the time. Techniques have been developed to minimize the infection. In a study in *Critical Care Medicine* by Bilen et al in April 1991 (24), an anti-bacterial vitacuff which resides at the insertion site was assessed. This device saved approximately $742.00 per patient, 10.5 physician hours, 14.0 nurse hours and 4.7 radiology hours, in terms of follow-up chest x-rays. Techniques to minimize infection also include dyed wire exchange, if there has been emergent insertion of a catheter, malfunction of the line, CVP to pulmonary artery catheter interconversions and/or positive blood cultures (Eyer *et. al.*, Critical Care Medicine, October 1990) (56). If there is purulent drainage at the skin site or cellulitis at the entry site, and/or a positive quantitative skin culture at 24 hours, then the line should be inserted at a new site.

At our institution, we reviewed the complications related to 600 Swan-Ganz catheter insertions (171). We had a 13% incidence of related sepsis, 2% incidence of congestive heart failure and a 0% incidence of pulmonary artery puncture. Our study demonstrated a 1.16% incidence of subclavian vein thrombosis, 1% incidence of pneumothorax and a 2% incidence of myocardial infarction, which may not have been related to the catheter insertion or maintenance but to the general medical condition of the patient.

GENERAL SYSTEMIC ISSUES IN NEUROVASCULAR CRITICAL CARE SEIZURES AND HEAD INJURY PATIENTS

Post-traumatic seizures are generally classified into three groups according to the time of their occurrence:

1) immediate seizures occur within the first 24 hours after the ictus with the majority occurring in the first several hours after admission;
2) delayed early seizures occur during the remainder of the first week;
3) late seizures are defined as those occurring greater than one week after the ictus (15).

Jennett and co-workers have termed the first two categories early and they are considered by him to be reactions to the acute event (90). He defines late seizures as unprovoked occurrences that are considered to be epileptic in nature.

Early seizures as defined have an incidence of approximately 1.9% in civilian head injuries, and 4.6% in consecutive admissions to a trauma center. The late seizure rate as defined is approximately 1.6% in the series of Annegers *et. al.* (15), and 5% in the series of Jennett (90).

The main risk factor for early seizures is an anatomical lesion, such as brain contusion or intracranial hematoma, be it epidural, subdural or subarachnoid. Jennett and co-workers indicated that 25% of patients with intracranial hematoma had early post-traumatic seizure activity. However, other investigators have found a lower incidence of approximately 19%. In the pediatric population, Hahn and co-workers found an increased rate of approximately 32% in children with subdural hematomas (76).

A great deal of controversy exists in the literature with regard to prophylaxis against seizure activity. There have been seven randomized double blind studies which have attempted to study the effectiveness of Phenytoin or Phenobarbital for preventing post-traumatic seizure activity. The studies of McQueen *et. al.* (127,128), Temkin *et. al.* (222) and Young *et. al.* (242) indicate that early treatment with Phenytoin prevents late seizures; however, the study of Loch reports a reduction of approximately 75%.

Short-term prophylaxis for one to two weeks was shown to reduce the occurrence of early post-traumatic seizures. In the study performed by Temkin and Young, the data available supports a short-term but not a long-term effect of the most commonly used drug, Phenytoin (210,222). A decision to use prophylaxis must include degree of pathology present, and the likelihood that the proposed treatment will substantially reduce the risk of in-hospital complications. There is ample evidence of the negative side effects of these anticonvulsants. Idiosyncratic reactions, such as rashes, are common in all studies. One study indicated a negative neuro-behavioral effect of Phenytoin in severe cases at one month after the injury, and in all later cases, evidence of improvement in the Phenytoin group when the drug was withdrawn (48).

When administered, Phenytoin is generally given in doses of 300-400 milligrams daily, either orally or parenterally. This follows a loading dose of approximately 1000 mg, which may be administered intravenously over 30 minutes with cardiac monitoring for arrhythmias. The second drug is Phenobarbital, which is generally given in doses of 90-120 mg daily. Status epilepticus may be treated with intravenous Diazapam in doses of 5-10 mg increments parenterally.

RESPIRATORY COMPLICATIONS

Pulmonary Complications

Pulmonary complications are the most devastating co-occurrences in the patient with a severe head injury and severe SAH (130,203). It is beyond the scope of this chapter to cover all pulmonary problems associated with head injury; however, several excellent reviews are available for the interested reader (16,21,44,49,83,91,92,152). Approximately 30% of patients with severe head injury (i.e. Glascow coma score of 8 or less on admission, having an associated PAO_2 less than 60 mm Hg on arrival to hospital. After initial management and admission into the Intensive Care Unit, approximately two-thirds of patients develop abnormalities on the chest x-ray at 72 hours. It has also been verified that patients who are hypercapnic or hypoxemic on admission are twice as likely to have a poor outcome.

Abnormal Respiratory Patterns

Cheyne-Stokes respiration, dyspnea, irregular breathing and periodic breathing are respiratory patterns commonly seen in patients with altered levels of consciousness (145). Dyspnea (less than 25 breaths per minute) is the only of the above patterns which have been associated with a poor outcome. This is particularly true when this pattern of breathing is associated with spontaneous hyperventilation (PCO_2 less than 30). This particular pattern of breathing has not been demonstrated to occur with any specific anatomic side of brain damage.

Reflexes to control the airways such as swallowing, gag and cough are either accurately suppressed or absent in patients with an altered level of consciousness. Frequently, vomiting occurs at the site of the accident with a resultant aspiration and pneumonia.In one study, 20% of patients admitted to an institution after a serious head injury had evidence of pulmonary aspiration (42). Although it is common practice to treat routinely with antibiotics and steroids, when aspiration is present, there have been no studies that have proven that this is efficacious (72,203).

Neurogenic Pulmonary Edema

During the Vietnam conflict, it was noted that approximately 85% of patients who died of severe injury had pathological evidence of pulmonary edema. This strengthened the hypothesis that massive cerebral injury alone in the absence of pulmonary trauma can result in massive pulmonary edema and hypoxemia (51,223,224). The pathogenesis is not well understood, however, many investigators propose that the acute cerebral insult leads to massive alpha-adrenergic over-stimulation and output with subsequent transient systemic and pulmonary vasoconstriction, and shifts the fluid into the pulmonary interstitium with associated massive increase in pulmonary venous pressures.

The incidence of neurogenic pulmonary edema varies in the literature from 0.1% to 85%. The presence of neurogenic pulmonary edema is often associated with a fatal outcome, and therefore must be a diagnosis of exclusion. Treatment of this condition centers on lowering the intracranial pressure and pulmonary support with standard measures such as peep, high frequency jet ventilation and diuresis if the patient is hemodynamically stable.

THE EFFECT OF PEEP ON INTRACRANIAL PRESSURE

It is well known that positive end expiratory pressure (PEEP) is an excellent method to increase the arterial oxygenation in patients with either noncardiogenic or cardiogenic pulmonary edema. It is recommended whenever systemic or arterial oxygenation requires greater than or equal to 60% O2 concentration to maintain PO2 greater than 60 mm Hg. PEEP increases oxygenation byreinflation of previously collapsed alveoli and/or under-ventilated areas increasing blood flow to ventilation ratios in these areas. It is believed that the functional residual capacity may be reduced in head injured patients that have normal chest x-rays, and at the commencement of PEEP may increase PO2 in patients without radiographic or physiologic evidence of pulmonary edema.

The role of PEEP in elevating intracranial pressure remains unclear. It is well known that intrathoracic pressure increases as well as central venous pressure, thereby, theoretically impeding venous return from the brain (40-42,197). Therefore ICP, theoretically, could increase dramatically in patients who have poor or reduced compliance. There have also been an equal number of studies that indicate that PEEP does not dramatically increase intracranial pressure in head injured victims. It is important that the patient's head be kept elevated at 30-60 degrees, and that the ideal head position be determined for each patient. With this simple maneuver, the ICP may remain stable even though the CVP becomes increased with the use of positive pressure. Most importantly, the cardiac output and index must be followed closely with the use of right heart catheters as a decrease in cardiac output with a resultant decrease in cerebral blood flow, may exacerbate a secondary injury of ischemia through marginal cerebral perfusion pressures.

In general, PEEP pressures of less than 10 cm H2O will not dramatically increase the ICP. The average change is approximately one mm Hg per 10 cm H2O of PEEP. Obviously, close observation is in order, and it is also important to remember that the ICP may increase when PEEP is discontinued abruptly such that appropriate weaning should be carried out in decrements of 2-5 cm H_2O (33).

COMMON PULMONARY COMPLICATIONS IN SAH AND HEAD INJURED PATIENTS

There are many causes of hypoxemia in a patient who has experienced a subarachnoid hemorrhage. Most common is atelectasis owing to the reduced lung volume demonstrated in head injured victims. There is less support for alveolar structures. It can be minimized by applying 3-5 sighs per hour to the patient on controlled ventilation. Endotracheal tube placement must also be adequately assessed as it should remain at least 4-6 cm above carina. In addition, inspissation of secretion is also a common problem which can be dealt with by maximal hydration and warming of the ventilatory gases. Aspiration, bacterial pneumonia, barotrauma, and ARDS are other common causes of hypoxemia in this patient population. It is beyond the scope of this discussion to cover the details of such syndromes, however, the reader is referred to several key references (16,21,49,50,153).

NEUROPHYSIOLOGICAL MONITORING IN THE NICU

New technologies have evolved which allow monitoring of electrocerebral function as well as cerebral blood flow and other sophisticated parameters; however, it should be remembered that the neurological exam is still the cornerstone of assessment and outcome. The Glascow Coma Score is commonly used in all neurosurgical intensive care units to assess day-to-day function as well as to predict prognosis in following daily progress for neurological improvement or deterioration.

Objective methods of monitoring such as the electroencephalogram, evoked potentials (consisting of somatosensory evoked potentials, brainstem auditory evoked potentials and visual evoked potentials) as well as cerebral blood flow monitoring have become routine in our unit. Their indications, methodology and pitfalls will be discussed briefly.

For many decades, the electroencephalogram or E.E.G. has been the cornerstone for objective monitoring of electrocerebral function

(156,198,215,219).   Different E.E.G. patterns have been described which delineate different types of coma, however, they have significant pitfalls when subjected to alterations of body temperature and in the presence of pharmocological agents. In the modern neurosurgical intensive care unit, the E.E.G. serves two prime functions: to determine the presence or absence of seizure activity, and secondly, to determine if adequate levels of Pentobarbital are being administered as evidenced by a burst suppression pattern. This is demonstrated as bursts of electrical activity interspersed with periods of electrocerebral silence. In general, adequate Pentobarbital suppression allows 6 bursts per minute with electrocerebral silence interspersed.   Evoked potentials are of three types: those produced by optical stimulation (VER's), by auditory stimulation (BAER's), and by cutaneous nerve stimulation assessing dorsal column function, termed somatosensory evoked potentials (SSEP's). These potentials are extremely small in amplitude as measured in microvolts and require computer averaging to sort them out from spontaneous or background noise (68,96). They are extremely useful in terms of monitoring to assess the current status of brain stem function in each selective patient. However, their use in diagnosis and prognosis of head injury is controversial (70,113,116,117,176). In general, it is the cortical component of the SSEP and VER which is evaluated. However, the cortical peak is extremely sensitive to alterations in body temperature as well as the presence of barbiturates. These modalities are not useful in determining brain stem function. However, brain stem auditory evoked responses are exquisitely sensitive in assessing the status of brain stem function, and are not as affected by alterations in body temperature (159). In addition, the five waves normally generated within the brain stem, if absent, are useful as criteria in determining brain death even in the presence of Pentobarb coma (231). Our current recommendations are that if a patient continues to have intractable intracranial pressure for 48 hours, we perform brainstem auditory evoked responses at 12 hour intervals. Two consecutive assessments with no brain stem activity on the BAER are indicative of brain death, and are used as legal criteria in the State of Pennsylvania. This dramatically simplifies matters in the face of Pentobarb coma or hypothermia, as the neurological exam and electroencephalogram are null and void (refer to Figure 6 and Figure 7).

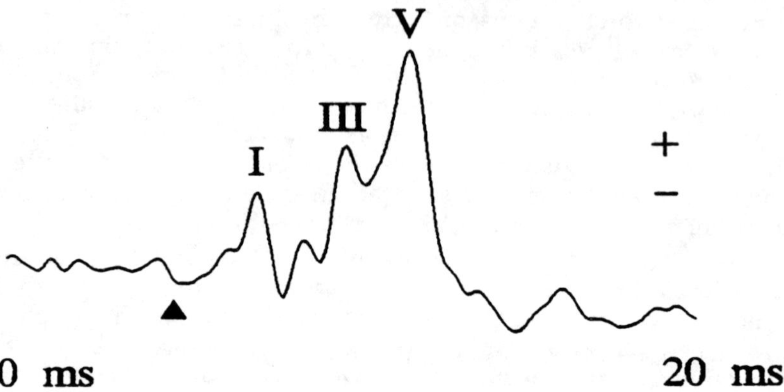

Figure 6.

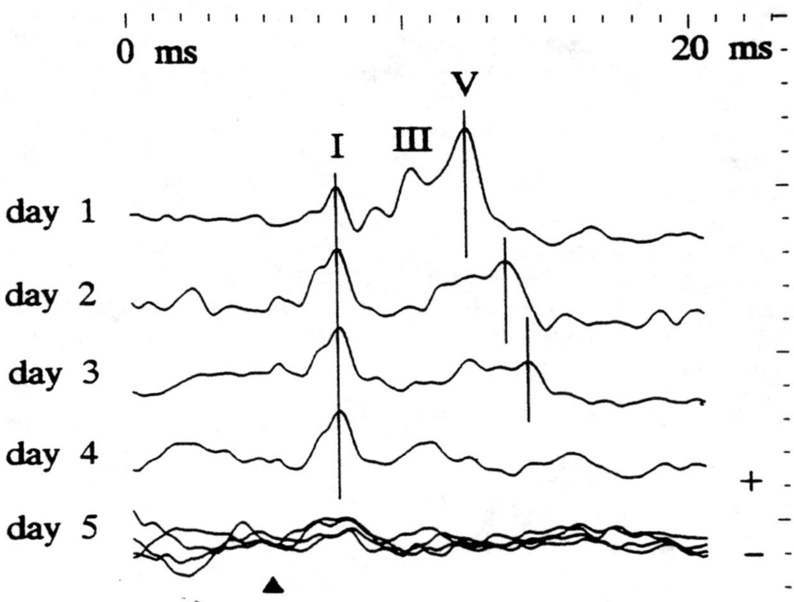

Figure 7.

MONITORING OF CEREBRAL BLOOD FLOW IN THE NICU

Cerebral blood flow was originally monitored by the Kety-Schmidt method in 1945, by use of nitrous oxide washout method. This was later modified with inhalational Xenon by Obrist in 1967 with external probe detectors over each hemisphere (109,147). Currently there are three other technologies available which can be used with relative ease in the neurosurgical intensive care area. One of the systems involves thermal diffusion technology, and the second is laser doppler technology, both of which are commercially available. Both of these require a small craniotomy for placement and are placed on the cortical surface of the brain if the patient has had a surgical procedure. A non-invasive indirect measurement of blood flow is by use of the transcranial doppler. This technique measures blood flow velocity, and its most useful role is in determining post-traumatic cerebral vasospasm, which will be discussed in a later section.

Questions remain about the prognostic value of cerebral blood flow in head injury victims and SAH (31,32,58,69,111). Extremes of high and low CBF have been associated with poor neurological outcome, with a blood flow value of less than 20cc/100 gm/minute almost always being associated with a poor neurological outcome. Langfitt and co-workers observed that an early reduction in cerebral blood flow returned to normal signified recovery, however, it continued to decrease in patients who ultimately succumbed from their injury. Some studies have documented that markedly elevated cerebral blood flow values have also been associated with poor neurological outcome (230).

In our unit, we routinely monitor cerebral blood flow using the thermal diffusion technique. The general values of flows which have been gained from experimental models of cerebral ischemia indicate normal flow values are approximately 40-60 cc/100gm/minute. It is a known fact that the level of consciousness becomes markedly altered, and that the electroencephalogram becomes suppressed with reduced amplitude and voltage when the CBF drops below 25cc/100gm/minute. The E.E.G. also becomes isoelectric at flow values of 18-20cc/100gm/minute (218). This can be a useful corollary when combined with barbiturate coma as flow values decrease presumably from decreased metabolic demand as the result of the Pentobarbital.

Flow probes are brought out through the scalp in a fashion similar to the ventriculostomy, and after 72 to 96 hours, the possibility of infection increases dramatically , and we therefore attempt to remove them during this time frame. After the blood flow probes have been removed, we then follow transcranial doppler velocities. Normal velocity ranges (anywhere from 50-80 cm/second, and values above 150 cm/second) are clearly related to reduced arterial diameter and possibly post-traumatic cerebral vasospasm. The important point is not the absolute value, but the change from the patient's own baseline reading, plus trend differences. If the patient has a baseline velocity of 50-80 cm/second, and then elevates to 100-150 cm/second, we will consider this patient to possibly have post-traumatic cerebral vasospasm, and therefore guide our fluid therapy so that euvolemia is achieved and maintained. It is extremely detrimental to have the patient's volume depleted either in the face of barbiturate therapy or in the face of post-traumatic cerebral vasospasm, as this can potentiate secondary ischemic injury. The absolute utility of direct and indirect measurements of cerebral blood flow is still under investigation, and its use cannot be absolutely recommended. We do find it useful in guiding the patient's intravascular volume, and as an indirect measurement of intact auto-regulation by comparing CO_2 reactivity to cerebral blood flow values.

FLUIDS AND ELECTROLYTES

In patients with either open or closed head injury, there is increased autonomic activity with constriction of renal arterioles, causing decreased urine output and salt retention. Stress hormone production is increased in terms of ACTH, endogenous glucocorticoids, and aldosterone, which further increase water retention that exceeds sodium retention. Water intoxication may develop with resultant dilutional hyponatremia, reduced serum osmolality, and exacerbation of cerebral edema. Many neurosurgeons continue to treat patients with head injury with fluid restriction; however, dilutional hyponatremia with a normal circulating blood volume can be avoided by administration of hypertonic salt solutions, in terms of 3-5% saline, with concomitant administration of low doses of furosemide which will excrete water in excess of salt. In the neurosurgical setting, hyponatremia has a different definition; serum sodiums of 130 are a major concern, whereas in the general medical patient or trauma patient, sodiums of 120-125 are easily tolerated. InCNS dysfunction, control of ICP and seizures becomes a major issue, and is much more difficult to treat at relatively lower reductions of serum sodium. In addition, hypomagnesemia will potentiate CNS irritability with resultant seizure activity, potentially exacerbating the secondary CNS trauma, previously discussed. Fluid and electrolyte disturbances, particularly the syndrome of inappropriate secretion of antidiuretic hormone (SIADH) and diabetes insipidus (DI) will be discussed briefly.

Water balance is primarily controlled by the posterior pituitary hormone known as vasopressin or antidiuretic hormone (ADH). This hormone is produced in the anterior hypothalamus and carried to the posterior pituitary gland, where it is secreted and carried to the renal system. There it is known to act on distal tubules to allow for retention of free water. In head injury, this balance may often be disturbed as a result of increased secretion of ADH. This syndrome results in retention of water and hyponatremia, defined as a sodium below 134 meq per liter. Hyponatremia often presents as deterioration in the level of consciousness, and as mentioned previously, can precipitate seizure activity. Diagnostic criteria for SIADH include normal renal function and adrenal function, serum osmolality of less than 280 milliosmoles per liter, high urine osmolality, and high urinary sodium secretion of greater than 25 meq per liter. This assumes that the patient is not receiving constant diuretic medications. Therapy of SIADH consists of mild fluid restriction, if indicated, although we prefer administration of hypertonic sodium 3% with associated furosemide administration.

Diabetes insipidus is different in its mechanism, in that it is usually due to trauma to the pituitary hypothalamic axis, with resultant loss of vasopressin production. Presenting symptoms are polyuria and polydipsia, particularly in the awake patient. Urine output may exceed 15 liters per day, with an associated low concentration with specific gravity generally below 1003. Hypernatremia often develops and is defined as a serum sodium greater than 125 meq per liter. Severe hypernatremia with a severe free water deficit often results. Aqueous vasopressin may be administered in doses of 2.5 to 5 units, every 4 to 6 hours, if the urine output remains at 200 - 300 ml per hour and serum sodium continues to be elevated. Replacement solution is generally 5% dextrose and water, and hyperglycemia may be treated with insulin administration if indicated.

NUTRITIONAL SUPPORT

In the past, little attention was given to the nutritional requirements of head injured patients. Although these patients often have an intact gastrointestinal tract, they often develop an ileus from impaired hypothalamic function (175). Enteral feeding has often been delayed for several days and this, combined with fluid restriction as has been practiced in the past, complicated the use of intravenous hyperalimentation (64). With trends changing concerning fluid management in head injury, early parenteral hyperalimentation is being used more in many intensive care units.

In comparison to the polytrauma patient, burn patients and septic patients, the increase in resting metabolic expenditure (RME) found in patients with open and closed head injuries is not overtly high, and is usually equivalent to the values reported in patients who are 30% burns, multiple trauma victims, and patients who are severely septic. In some studies of patients with head injury, higher values of RME (1.7 to 1.8 times those expected) were found for long periods of time, reflecting that some head injury patients have an RME equivalent to that of patients with 40-50% burns (64). The extent of nitrogen excretion in relation to the increase in RME was higher than the values reported for any group of injured patients, resulting in a percent of calories consumed (PCC) of approximately 24%. A PCC of greater than 20% has been reported in very critical patients, particularly burn, sepsis and trauma. In the past, steroids, particularly dexamethasone, were administered to open and closed head injuries. It is possible that the extreme nitrogen loss found in these earlier studies was related to the medication. Currently, new data is being evaluated by many investigators to determine if nitrogen loss is markedly decreased in the absence of the steroid administration.

Several studies have indicated that massive nitrogen excretion may occur up to ranges of 25 grams per day, or 338 mg/Kg per day. Increases in caloric expenditure from 120 - 270% of basal metabolic rate (BMR) have been observed (107,229). Studying prospectively head injured patients up to 10 days following insult, Long and co-workers observed a mean peak 24 hour caloric expenditure of 160% of BMR. This peak occurred between day 5 and day 8 in all patients whom they studied. Many other studies have verified their findings. Currently, we are very aggressive in beginning early total parenteral nutrition in head injured patients and poor grade SAH patients (above grade 3). Immediately postoperatively, a solution of 25% dextrose and 4.25% amino acids is begun as a constant infusion. The rate of infusion is increased over a three to four day period, up to 3,000 ml per day, providing 20.4 grams of nitrogen and 2650 kilocalories per day. In addition, we have increased the caloric input by the administration of 500 ml of intralipid, providing an additional caloric intake of 510 kilocalories per day. Problems with parenteral nutrition are primarily hyperglycemia, which is known to be associated with increased carbon dioxide production and oxygen consumption. In addition, there is preliminary experimental data which indicates that hyperglycemia may potentiate cerebral ischemic injury by increasing lactic acid production (155,190,191). We maintain very tight control of the serum glucose, maintaining it at levels of less than or equal to 200 mg %. Insulin may be added to the feedings as indicated.

Once the ileus has passed, we institute enteral feedings, generally through a small bore nasogastric or nasoduodenal tube. To minimize complications in terms of aspiration, the rate and concentration of the feeding solution are increased slowly, the gastric content is aspirated every six hours and the patient's head is kept elevated at greater than or equal to 30 degrees. Many products are available, such as Ensure and Osmolyte, which provide 1 calorie per cc and 38 grams of protein per liter. The concentration and rate are increased progressively over a one week period, to provide a maximum intake of 1.5 to 2 grams of protein per kilogram per day and 2500 to 3000 kilocalories. Lomotil may be administered if diarrhea becomes a problem. Water and electrolyte balances, as well as potassium administration, can be performed parenterally to supplement electrolyte balance.

EXTRACRANIAL COMPLICATIONS

Extracranial complications of the patient with subarachnoid and head injury include pneumonia, sinus infections, deep venous thrombosis, pulmonary embolism, ARDS and gastrointestinal complications.

PNEUMONIA

Pneumonia is currently the primary cause of fatal non-succumbent infections in intensive care units in the United States, and are primarily related to gram negative infections (152). Colonization of the nasal and oral pharynx occurs in up to 45% of ICU patients (91,92). Respiratory tract infections develop in approximately 25% of those who are colonized. The most common organisms isolated include pseudomonas aeruginosa, anaerobe bacterial species, E coli and Klebsiella pneumonia. Route of infection is generally aspiration in patients who have abnormal cough and swallowing reflexes. In addition they are often receiving medications such as Pentobarb, which reduces the ability to fight infection. The interested reader is referred to other references for an in-depth review.

When a source of fever can not be determined one must also consider sinusitis in patients with head injury (35). It is most commonly seen when the patient has had prolonged nasotracheal or nasogastric tubes in place and in general requires no additional treatment other than removal of these devices. Gram negative organisms are most commonly recovered when sinusitis of this nature is encountered. The diagnosis is easily made on reviewing CT scans which have been performed for other reasons.

DEEP VENOUS THROMBOSIS
AND PULMONARY EMBOLISM

In victims of trauma, the reported incidence of pulmonary embolus is anywhere from 4 to 22% (195). The incidence of deep venous thrombosis is 20 to 90%. Patients with neurological injuries are often immobilized for long periods of time and are therefore at increased risk. The most reliable method of detecting DVT is venography and for pulmonary embolus, pulmonary angiography. Often times doppler ultrasonography of the lower extremities may be accurate in 80% of the cases. Ventilation perfusion scans have similar figures in diagnosing pulmonary embolus and can be obtained quicker and with less morbidity than a pulmonary angiogram.

In a patient with a head injury or SAH, the problem is one of treatment. Heparin is usually contraindicated when intracranial blood is present and therefore the use of vena cava filters is often recommended in the acute phase. Prophylaxis is extremely important in terms of pneumatic compression stockings. Prophylactic heparin again should not be used in the patient with intracranial blood or other injuries where anti-coagulation would be contraindicated. Shackford and co-workers reported that 14% of trauma victims could not receive mechanical or anticoagulant prophylaxis because of their associated injuries (195).

GASTROINTESTINAL COMPLICATIONS

The reported incidence of erosive gastritis in head injured victims and critically ill SAH patients is approximately 74 to 100% (30,93,94,110,146). 80% of patients admitted to an intensive care unit with a diagnosis of head injury experienced some degree of gastrointestinal hemorrhage within the first week. The etiology of erosive gastritis and ulceration is controversial; however, hyperacidity is thought to be a major culprit. The incidence of erosive gastritis does not seem to correlate with the degree of head injury and intracranial hypertension (95). There are investigators who believe that ischemia of the gastric mucosa may play an equally important role in the development of this problem. Prophylaxis against gastrointestinal hemorrhage has been routine in most intensive care settings through the use of antacids and H2 blockers in an attempt to raise the pH and reduce the risk of hemorrhage. This maneuver may lead to bacterial colonization of the stomach with a greater risk for bacterial pneumonia secondary to aspiration of gastric contents (65,148). Perhaps by maintaining normal intravascular volume and blood pressure in the avoidance of systemic vasoconstrictors, gastric mucosal ischemia may be avoided with complications previously outlined.

DISORDERS OF COAGULATION

Approximately 40-70% of patients with either open or closed head injury have been shown to have abnormal clotting factors, and either clinical or subclinical coagulopathy (38,102). The incidence in SAH has not well been worked out, however patients with sever ICH have also been observed to have abnormal coagulation profiles. This has been related to release of large quantities of brain thromboplastin into the circulation and activation of the coagulation profile. The incidence of coagulation disorder, secondary to head injuries is directly proportional to the severity of the head injury, according to numerous authors. In the study of Sande and Vandervelkamps, the incidence of abnormalities in coagulation was directly related to the level of consciousness and brain stem function (180). Almost all of their patients with Glasgow Coma Score of less than 8 had abnormal coagulation tests. If DIC does develop in the neurosurgical patient, treatment is similar to the treatment of DIC in damage to other organ systems; however, one is extremely reluctant to treat with Heparin in the perioperative period after neurosurgical injury. Replacement therapy is given in terms of fresh frozen plasma and platelet concentrates, although the argument has been made that blood component administration may potentiate the DIC cascade (102).

REFERENCES

1.　　Aaslid, R., P. Huber, and H. Nornes, transcranial Doppler method in the evaluation of cerebrovascular spasm. *Neuroradiology.* 28:11-16, 1986.

2.　　Aaslid, R., K.F. Lindegaard, W. Sorteberg, and H. Nornes, Cerebral autoregulation dynamics in humans. *Stroke.* 20:45-52, 1989.

3.　　Aaslid, R., D.W. Newell, R. Stooss, W. Sorteberg, and K.F. Lindegaard, Assessment of cerebral autoregulation dynamics from simultaneous arterial and venous transcranial Doppler recordings in humans. *Stroke.* 22:1148-1154, 1991.

4.　　Adams, H.P., Jr. Early management of the patient with recent aneurysmal subarachnoid hemorrhage. *Stroke.* 17:1068-1070, 1986.

5.　　Adams, H.P., Jr., D.D. Jergenson, N.F. Kassell, A.L. and Sahs, Pitfalls in the recognition of subarachnoid hemorrhage. *JAMA* 244:794-796, 1980.

6.　　Adams, H.P., Jr., N.F. Kassell, G.A. Kongable, and J.C. Torner, Intracranial operation within seven days of aneurysmal subarachnoid hemorrhage. Results in 150 patients. *Arch Neurol* 45:1065-1069, 1988.

7.　　Adams, H.P., Jr., N.F. Kassell, J.C. Torner, and E.C. Haley Jr., Predicting cerebral ischemia after aneurysmal subarachnoid hemorrhage: influences of clinical condition, CT results, and antifibrinolytic therapy. A report of the Cooperative Aneurysm Study. *Neurology.* 37:1586-1591, 1987.

8.　　Adams, H.P., Jr., N.F. Kassell, J.C. Torner, D.W. Nibbelink, and A.L. Sahs, Early management of aneurysmal subarachnoid hemorrhage. A report of the Cooperative Aneurysm Study. *J Neurosurg* 54:141-145, 1981.

9.　　Adams, H.P., N.F. Kassell, J.C. Torner, and A.L. Sahs, CT and clinical correlations in recent aneurysmal subarachnoid hemorrhage: a preliminary report of the Cooperative Aneurysm Study. *Neurology.* 33:981-988, 1983.

10.　　Adams, H.P., Jr., D.W. Nibbelink, J.C. Torner, A.L. and Sahs, Antifibrinolytic therapy in patients with aneurysmal subarachnoid hemorrhage. A report of the cooperative aneurysm study. *Arch Neurol* 38:25-29, 1981.

11.　　Adams, H.P., Jr. and A.L. Sahs, Aneurysmal subarachnoid hemorrhage. *Mod. Concepts. Cardiovasc. Dis* 50:49-54, 1981.

12.   Alafaci, C., I. Jansen, M.A. Arbab, Y. Shiokawa, N.A. Svendgaard, and L. Edvinsson, Enhanced vasoconstrictor effect of endothelin in cerebral arteries from rats with subarachnoid hemorrhage. *Acta Physiol Scand* 138:317-319, 1990.

13.   Albers, G.W., M.P. Goldberg, and D.W. Choi, N-methl-D-aspartate antagonists: Ready for clinical trial in brain ischemia? *Ann Neurol* 25:398-390, 1989.

14.   Ando, T., N. Sakai, H. Yamada, et al. Analysis of reruptured cerebral aneurysms and the prophylactic effects of barbiturate therapy on the early stage. *Neurol Res.* 11:245-248, 1989.

15.   Annegers, J.F., J.D. Grabow, R.V. Groover, and et al, Seizures after head trauma: A population study. *Neurology* 30:683-689, 1980.

16.   Arms, R.A., D.E. Dines, and T.C. Tinstman, Aspiration pneumonia. *Chest* 65:136-130, 1974.

17.   Astrup, J., P.M. Sorenesn, and H.R. Sorenesn, Inhibition of cerebral oxygen and glucose consumption in the dog by hypothermia, pentobarbital, and lidocaine. *Anesthesiology* 55:263-260, 1981.

18.   Auer, L.M. Acute operation and preventive nimodipine improve outcome in patients with ruptured cerebral aneurysms. *Neurosurgery.* 15:57-66, 1984.

19.   Auer, L.M., Brandt, L., Ebeling, U., et al. Nimodipine and early aneurysm operation in good condition SAH patients. *Acta Neurochir* 82:7-13, 1986.

20.   Awad, I.A., Carter, L.P., Spetzler, R.F., Medina, M. and Williams, F.C., Jr. Clinical vasospasm after subarachnoid hemorrhage: response to hypervolemic hemodilution and arterial hypertension. *Stroke.* 18:365-372, 1987.

21.   Baigelman, W. and J.C. O'Brien, Pulmonary effects of head trauma. *Neurosurg.* 9:729-740, 1981.

22.   Bell, B.A., M.A. Smith, C.M. Kean, and et al, Brain water measured by magnetic resonance imaging. *Lancet* 1:66-60, 1987.

23.   Benveniste, H. The excitotoxin hypothesis in relation to cerebral ischemia. *Cerebrovasc. Brain Metab Rev* 3:213-245, 1991.

24.   Bilen, Z., P.F. Weinberg, Y. Gowani, I.L. Cohen, S. Socaris, I.A. Fein, Clinical utility and cost -effectiveness of protective sleeve pulmonary artery catheters. *Crit. Care Med* 19:491-496, 1991.

25.   Bohrer, H. and F. Fleischer, Errors in biochemical and haemodynamic data obtained using introducer lumen and proximal port of Swan Ganz catheter. *Intensive. Care.Med.* 15:330-331, 1989.

26.   Brandt, L., K.E. Andersson, B. Ljunggren, H. Saveland, T. and Ryman, Cerebrovascular and cerebral effects of nimodipine--an update. *Acta Neurochir.Suppl.* 45:11-20, 1988.

27.   Brandt, L., B. Ljunggren, H. Saveland, K.E. Andersson, and E. Vinge, Cerebral vasospasm and calcium channel blockade. Nimodipine treatment in patients with aneurysmal subarachnoid hemorrhage. *Acta Pharmacol. Toxicol.* 58 Suppl 2:151-155, 1986.

28.   Brandt, L., H. Saveland, B. Romner, and T. Ryman, Does nimodipine eliminate arterial hypertension as a prognostic risk factor in subarachnoid hemorrhage? *Br J Neurosurg* 5:485-489, 1991.

29.   Braughler, J.M. and E.D. Hall, Central nervous system trauma and stroke. I. Biochemical considerations for oxygen radical formation and lipid peroxidation. *Journal of Free Radicals and Biological Medicine* 6:289-280, 1989.

30.   Brown, T.H., P.F. Davidson, and G.M. Larson, Acute gastritis occurring within 24 hours of severe head injury. *Gastrointest Endosc* 35:37-30, 1989.

31.   Bruce, D.A., A. Alavi, L. Bilaniuk, and et al, Diffuse cerebral swelling following head injuries in children: The syndrome of "malignant brain edema" *J Neurosurg* 54:170-178, 1981.

32.   Bruce, D.A., R.C. Raphaely, A.I.   Goldberg,   and et al, Pathophysiology, treatment, and outcome following severe head injury in children. *Child's Brain* 5:174-191, 1979.

33.   Burchiel, K.J., T.D. Steege, A.R. and Wyler, Intracranial pressure changes in brain injured patients requiring positive end-expiratory pressure ventilation. *Neurosurg.* 8:443-449, 1981.

34.   Burrows, G. Disorders of the Cerebral Circulation. London: Longman, 1846,

35.   Caplan, E.S. and N.J. Hoyt, Nosocomial sinusitis. *JAMA* 247:639-630, 1982.

36.   Carpenter, D.A., R.L. Grubb Jr., L.W. Tempel, and W.J. Powers, Cerebral oxygen metabolism after aneurysmal subarachnoid hemorrhage. *J Cereb Blood Flow Metab* 11:837-844, 1991.

37.   Chiang J., M. Kowada A. Ames A. III, Wright R.L., Majno G., Cerebral Ischemia III. Vascular Changes. *AM J Pathol* 52:455-476, 1968.

38.   Clark, J.A., R.E. Tinelli, and M.G. Metsky, Disseminated intravascular coagulation following cranial trauma. *J Neurosurg* 52:266-269, 1980.

39.   Colardyn, F., J. Vandenbogaerde, C. De Niel, and L. Jordaens, Ventricular pacing via a Swan Ganz catheter: a new mode of pacemaker therapy. *Acta Cardiol.* 41:23-29, 1986.

40.   Cooper, K.R. and P. Boswell, Reduced functional residual capacity and abnormal oxygenation in patients with severe head injury. *Chest* 84:29-35, 1983.

41.   Cooper, K.R. and P.A. Boswell, Safe use of PEEP in head injured patients. *J Neurosurg* 63:552-555, 1985.

42.   Cooper, K.R. and C.F. Morrow, Pulmonary complications associated with head injury. *Resp Care* 29:263-269, 1984.

43.   Cooper, P., S. Moody, W. Clark, and et al, Dexamethasone and severe head injury. A prospective double blind study. *J Neurosurg* 51:307-300, 1979.

44.   Craven, D.E. and K.A. Steger, Nosocomial pneumonia in the intubated patient. New concepts on pathogenesis and prevention. *Infect Dis Clin North Am* 3:843-840, 1989.

45.   D'Ambra, M.N., W. Dewhirst, M. Jacobs, B. Bergus, L. Borges, and A. Hilgenberg, Cross-clamping the thoracic aorta. Effect on intracranial pressure. *Circulation.* 78:III198-III202, 1988.

46.   Dearden, N.M., J.S. Gibson, D.G. McDowal, and et al, Effect of high-dose dexamethasone on outcome from severe head injury. *J Neurosurg* 64:81-80, 1986.

47.   Dearden, N.M. and J.D. Miller, Paired comparison of hypnotic and osmotic therapy in the reduction of intracranial hypertension after severe head injury. In: *Intracranial Pressure VII*, edited by Hoff, J.T. and Betz, A.L. Berlin: Springer-Verlag, 1989, p. 474-470.

48.   Dikmen, S.S., N.R. Temkin, B. Miller, and et al, Neurobehavioral effects of phenytoin prophylaxis of post-traumatic seizures. *JAMA* 265:1991.

49.   Donegan, M.F. and R.F. Bedford, Intravenously administered lidocaine prevents intracranial hypertension during endotracheal suctioning. *Anesthesiology* 52:516-510, 1980.

50.   Driks, M.R., D.E. Craven, and B.R. Celli, Nosocomial pneumonia in intubated patients given sucralfate as compared with antacids or histamine type 2 blockers. *N Engl J Med* 317:1376-1370, 1987.

51.   Ducker, T.B. and R. Simmons, Increased ICP and pulmonary edema. Hemodynamic response of dogs and monkeys to raised intracranial pressure. *J Neurosurg* 28:118-123, 1968.

52.   Eisenberg, H., R. Frankowski, C. Contant, C. and et al, High-dose barbiturate control of elevated intracranial pressure in patients with severe head injury. *J Neurosurg* 69:15-10, 1988.

53.   Espinosa, F., B. Weir, T. Overton, W. Castor, M. Grace, and D.A. Boisvert, Randomized placebo-controlled double-blind trial of nimodipine after SAH in monkeys. Part 1: Clinical and radiological findings. *J Neurosurg* 60:1167-1175, 1984.

54.   Espinosa, F., B. Weir, T. Shnitka, T. Overton, and D. A. Boisvert, Randomized placebo-controlled double-blind trial of nimodipine after SAH in monkeys. Part 2: Pathological findings. *J Neurosurg* 60:1176-1185, 1984.

55.   Evans, D.E. and A.I. Kobrine, Reduction of experimental intracranial hypertension by lidocaine. *Neurosurg.* 20:542-540, 1987.

56.   Eyer, S., C. Brummitt, K. Crossley, R. Siegal, and F. Cerra, Catheter related sepsis:prospective, randomized study of three methods of long-term catheter maintenance. *Crit. Care Med.* 18:1073-1079, 1990.

57.   Faden, A.I., P. Demediuk, S.S. Panter, and et al, The role of excitatory amino acids and NMDA receptors in traumatic brain injury. *Science* 244:798-790, 1989.

58.   Fieschi, C., N. Battistini, A. Beduschi, and et al, Regional cerebral blood flow and intraventricular pressure in acute head injuries. *J Neurol Neurosurg Psychiatry* 37:1378-1388, 1974.

59.   Fischer EG, A. Ames III. Studies on mechanisms of impairment of cerebral circulation following ischemia: effect of hemodilution and perfusion pressure. *Stroke* 3:538-542, 1972.

60.   Fisher, A.B. Intracellular production of oxygen-derived free radicals. In: *Oxygen Radicals and Tissue Injury*, edited by Halliwell, B. Bethesda: Federation of American Societies for Experimental Biology, 1988, p. 34-30.

61.   Fisher, C.M., J.P. Kistler J.M. Davis, Relation of Cerebral Vasospasm to Subarachnoid Hemorrhage visualized by Computed Tomographic Scanning. *Neurosurgery* 6:1:1980.

62.   Flamm, E.S., H.P. Adams Jr., D.W. Beck, et al. Dose-escalation study of intravenous nicardipine in patients with aneurysmal subarachnoid hemorrhage. *J Neurosurg* 68:393-400, 1988.

63.   Fogliani, J., C. Armaghanian, J. Romeuf, M. and Rouge, [Method for prolonged hemodynamic and respiratory monitoring. I. Technical study involving 45 patients]. *Ann. Anesthesiol.Fr.* 22:581-591, 1981.

64.   Gadisseaux, D., J.P. Ward, H.F. Young, and et al, Nutrition and the neurosurgical patient. *Neurosurg.* 60:219-232, 1984.

65.   Giannella, R.A., S.A. Broitman, and N. Zamcheck, Gastric acid barrier to ingested microorganisms in man: Studies in vivo and in vitro. *Gut* 13:251-250, 1972.

66.   Giller, C.A. Transcranial Doppler monitoring of cerebral blood velocity during craniotomy. *Neurosurgery.* 25:769-776, 1989.

67.   Gilsbach, J.M. and A.G. Harders, Morbidity and mortality after early aneurysm surgery--a prospective study with nimodipine prevention. *Acta Neurochir* 96:1-7, 1989.

68.   Glaser, E.M. and D.S. Ruchkins, Basics of signal processing. In: *Principles of Neurobiological Signal Analysis*, edited by Glaser, E.M. and Ruchkin, D.S. New York: Academic Press, 1976, p. 55-102.

69.   Gobiet, G., W. Grote, and W.J. Bock, The relationship between intracranial pressure, mean arterial pressure and cerebral blood flow in patients with severe head injury. *Acta Neurochir (Wien)* 32:13-24, 1975.

70.   Goitein, K.J., P. Gainmesse, and H. Sohmer, The relationship between cerebral perfusion pressure and auditory nerve brain stem evoked response: Diagnostic and prognostic implications. In: *Intracranial Pressure V*, edited by Ishii, S., Nagai, H. and Brack, M. Berlin: Springer-Verlag, 1983, p. 468-473.

71.   Grant, P.K., R.B. Hopkinson, B. Kumar, S.P. Singh, and S. Reuben, Repeated percutaneous internal jugular cannulation using flow directed Swan Ganz catheter. *Intensive. Care. Med.* 10:293-295, 1984.

72.   Greenblatt, S.H., C.L. Foy, W.S. Blakemore, and et al, Catabolic effect of dexamethasone in patients with major head injury. *JPEN* 13:373-376, 1989.

73.   Grotenhuis, J.A. and W. Bettag, Prevention of symptomatic vasospasm after SAH by constant venous infusion of nimodipine. *Neurol Res.* 8:243-249, 1986.

74.   Grubb, R.L., Jr. and M.E. Raichle, Effects of hemorrhagic and pharmacologic hypotension on cerebral oxygen utilization and blood flow. *Anesthesiology.* 56:3-8, 1982.

75.   Gudeman, S., J. Miller, D. and Becker, Failure of high-dose steroid therapy to influence intracranial pressure in patients with severe head injury. *J Neurosurg* 51:301-300, 1979.

76.   Hahn, Y.S., C. Chyung, M.J. Barthel, J. Bailes, A.M. Flannery, and D.G. McLone, Head injuries in children under 36 months of age. Demography and outcome. *Childs. Nerv. Syst.* 4:34-40, 1988.

77.   Hall, E.D. and M. Braughler, The role of oxygen radical-induced lipid peroxidation in acute central nervous system trauma. In: *Oxygen Radicals and Tissue Injury*, edited by Halliwell, B. Bethesda: Federation of American Societies for Experimental Biology, 1988, p. 92-90.

78.   Hall, E.D., K.E. Pazara, and J.M. Braughler, 21-Aminosteroid lipid peroxidation inhibitor U74006F protects against cerebral ischemia in gerbils. *Stroke* 19:997-990, 1988.

79.   Hall, E.D. and M.A. Travis, Effects of the nonglucocorticoid 21-aminosteroid U74006F on acute cerebral hypoperfusion following experimental subarachnoid hemorrhage. *Exp. Neurol* 102:244-248, 1988.

80.   Hall, E.D. and P.A. Yonkers, Attenuation of postischemic cerebral hypoperfusion by the 21-aminosteroid U74006F. *Stroke* 19:340, 1988.

81.   Harders, A. and J. Gilsbach, Hemodynamic effectiveness of nimodipine on spastic brain vessels after subarachnoid hemorrhage evaluated by the transcranial Doppler method. A review of clinical studies. *Acta Neurochir Suppl.* 45:21-28, 1988.

82.   Harders, A.G. and J.M. Gilsbach, Time course of blood velocity changes related to vasospasm in the circle of Willis measured by transcranial Doppler ultrasound. *J Neurosurg* 66:718-728, 1987.

83.   Hemmer, M. Ventilatory support for pulmonary failure of the head trauma patient. *Bull Eur Physiopathol Respir* 21:287-293, 1985.

84.   Hongo, K., N.F. Kassell, T. Nakagomi, et al. Subarachnoid hemorrhage inhibition of endothelium-derived relaxing factor in rabbit basilar artery. *J Neurosurg* 69:247-253, 1988.

85.   Hubschmann, O.R. and D. Kornhauser, Effect of subarachnoid hemorrhage on the extracellular microenvironment. *J Neurosurg* 56:216-221, 1982.

86.   Hubschmann, O.R. and D.C. Nathanson, The role of calcium and cellular membrane dysfunction in experimental trauma and subarachnoid hemorrhage. *J Neurosurg* 62:698-703, 1985.

87.   Hutchison, K. and B. Weir, Transcranial Doppler studies in aneurysm patients. *Can. J Neurol Sci.* 16:411-416, 1989.

88.   Ilias, W., F. Lackner, and M. Zimpfer, [The intraoperative use of falipamil (AQ-A39), a new calcium antagonist with specific bradytropic properties]. *Anesthesist.* 39:487-492, 1990.

89.   Iwadate, Y., J. Ono, Y. Okimura, S. Suda, K. Isobe, and A. Yamaura, [Computed tomography in diagnosis of diffuse axonal injury]. *No. Shinkei. Geka.* 18:915-920, 1990.

90.   Jennett, B. *Epilepsy After Nonmissile Injuries*, Chicago:Year Book Medical Publishers Inc., 1975. Ed. 2nd

91.   Johanson, W.G., A.K. Pierce, J.P. and Sanford, Changing pharyngeal bacterial flora of hospitalized patients: Emergence of gram-negative bacilli. *N Engl J Med* 281:1137-1130, 1969.

92.   Johanson, W.G., A.K. Pierce, J.P. Sanford, and et al, Nosocomial respiratory infections with gram-negative bacilli: The significance of colonization of the respiratory tract. *Ann Intern Med* 77:701-700, 1972.

93.   Kamada, T., H. Fusamoto, S. Kawano, and et al, Gastrointestinal bleeding following head injury: A clinical study of 433 cases. *J Trauma* 17:44-40, 1977.

94.   Kamada, T., H. Fusamoto, S. Kawano, and et al, Acute gastroduodenal lesions in head injury. An endoscopic study. *Am J Gastroenterol* 68:249-240, 1977.

95.   Kamada, T., N. Sato, S. Kawano, and et al, Gastric mucosal hemodynamics after thermal or head injury. A clinical application of reflectance spectro-photometry. *Gastroenterology* 83:535-530, 1982.

96.   Kamath, M.V., S.N. Reddy, D.N. Ghista, and et al, Power spectral analysis of normal and pathological brainstem auditory evoked potentials. *Int J Biomed Comput* 21:33-54, 1987.

97.   Kanamaru, K., S. Waga, T. Kojima, K. Fujimoto, and S. Niwa, Endothelium-dependent relaxation of canine basilar arteries. Part 2: Inhibition by hemoglobin and cerebrospinal fluid from patients with aneurysmal subarachnoid hemorrhage. *Stroke.* 18:938-943, 1987.

98.   Kassell, N.F., H.P. Adams Jr., J.C. Torner, A.L. and Sahs, Influence of timing of admission after aneurysmal subarachnoid hemorrhage on overall outcome. Report of the cooperative aneurysm study. *Stroke*. 12:620-623, 1981.

99.   Kassell, N.F., D.J. Boarini, H.P. Adams Jr., et al. Overall management of ruptured aneurysm: comparison of early and late operation. *Neurosurgery*. 9:120-128, 1981.

100. Katayama, Y., D.P. Becker, T. Tamura, and et al, Massive increases in extracellular potassium and the indiscriminate release of glutamate following concussive brain injury. *J Neurosurg* 73:889-880, 1990.

101. Katayama, Y., M.K. Cheung, L. Gorman, and et al, Increase in extracellular glutamate and associated massive ionic fluxes following concussive brain injury. *Society for Neurosciences* 14:1154-1150, 1988.(Abstract)

102. Kaufman, H.H. Delayed and recurrent intracranial hematomas related to disseminated intravascular clotting and fibrinolysis in head injury. *Neurosurg*. 7:445-449, 1980.

103. Kellie, G. *Transactions of the Medico-Chirurgical Society of Edinburgh* 1:84-80, 1824.

104. Kim, K.H., H. Takeuchi, Y. Kamatani, H. Minakata, and K. Nomoto, Slow inward current induced by achatin-I, an endogenous peptide with a D-Phe residue. *Eur. J Pharmacol*. 194:99-106, 1991.

105. Kim, P., R.R. Lorenz, T.M. Sundt Jr. and P.M. Vanhoutte, Release of endothelium-derived relaxing factor after subarachnoid hemorrhage. *J Neurosurg* 70:108-114, 1989.

106. King, L.R., R.L. McLaurin, and H.C. Knowles, Acid-base balance and arterial and CSF lactate levels following human head injury. *J Neurosurg* 40:617-610, 1974.

107. Kolpek, J.H., L.G. Ott, K.E. Record, and et al, Comparison of urinary urea nitrogen excretion and measured energy expenditure in spinal cord injury and nonsteroid-treated severe head trauma patients. *JPEN* 13:277-280, 1989.

108. Krueger, C., B. Weir, M. Nosko, D. Cook, and S. Norris, Nimodipine and chronic vasospasm in monkeys: Part 2. Pharmacological studies of vessels in spasm. *Neurosurgery*. 16:137-140, 1985.

109. Langfitt, T., W.D. Obrist, T.A. Gennarelli, and et al, Correlation of cerebral blood flow with outcome in head-injured patients. *Ann Surg* 186:411-414, 1977.

110. Larson, G.M., S. Koch, T.M. O'Dorisio, and et al, Gastric response to severe head injury. *Am J Surg* 147:97-90, 1984.

111. Lassen, N.A. The luxury perfusion syndrome and its possible relation to acute metabolic acidosis localized within the brain. *Lancet* 2:1113-1114, 1966.

112. Leech, P. and J. Miller, Intracranial volume-pressure relationships during experimental brain compression in primates. 3. Effect of mannitol and hyperventilation. *J Neurol Neurosurg Psychiatry* 37:1015-1010, 1974.

113. Lesser, R.P, P. Raudzens, H. Luders, and et al, Postoperative neurological deficits may occur despite unchanged intraoperative somatosensory evoked potentials. *Ann Neurol* 19:22-25, 1986.

114. Levene, M.I., N.A. Gibson, A.C. Fenton, E. Papathoma, and D. Barnett, The use of a calcium-channel blocker, nicardipine, for severely asphyxiated newborn infants. *Dev. Med. Child. Neurol.* 32:567-574, 1990.

115. Lindegaard, K.F., H. Nornes, S.J. Bakke, W. Sorteberg, and P. Nakstad, Cerebral vasospasm after subarachnoid hemorrhage investigated by means of transcranial Doppler ultrasound. *Acta Neurochir Suppl.* 42:81-84, 1988.

116. Lindsay, K., A. Pasaoglu, D. Hirst, and et al, Somatosensory and auditory brain stem conduction after head injury: A comparison with clinical features in prediction of outcome. *Neurosurg* 26:278-285, 1990.

117. Lindsay, K.W., G.M. Teasdale, and R.P. Knill Jones, Observer variability in assessing the clinical features of subarachnoid hemorrhage. *J Neurosurg* 58:57-62, 1983.

118. Lundberg, N. Continuous recording and control of ventricular fluid pressure in neurosurgical practice. *Acta Psychiatr Neurol Scand* 36:1-193, 1960.

119. Maione, M., G.P. Fabbrini, C. Mazzi, P. Nannicini, and P. Grassi, [Septic shock in a case of purulent pericarditis. Usefulness of hemodynamic study with Swan-Ganz catheterization]. *Minerva. Anestesiol.* 55:329-330, 1989.

120. Marmarou, A., J.D. Anderson, H.M. Eisenberg, and et al, The traumatic coma data bank: Monitoring of ICP. In: *Intracranial Pressure VII*, edited by Hoff, J.T. and Betz, A.L. Berlin: Springer-Verlag, 1989, p. 549-540.

121. Marshall, L., J. King, and T. Langfitt, The complications of high-dose corticosteroid therapy in neurosurgical patients: A prospective study. *Ann Neurol* 1:201-200, 1977.

122. Marshall, L., R. Smith, L. Rauscher, and et al, Mannitol dose requirements in brain-injured patients. *J Neurosurg* 48:169-160, 1978.

123. Marshall, L.F. Treatment of brain swelling and brain edema in man. *Adv Neurol* 28:459-450, 1980.

124. Marzatico, F., P. Gaetani, G. Spanu, E. Buratti, and Rodriguez, Effects of nicardipine treatment on Na(+)-K+ ATPase and lipid peroxidation after experimental subarachnoid hemorrhage. *Acta Neurochir* 108:128-133, 1991.

125. Maset, A., A. Marmarou, J. Ward, and et al, Pressure-volume index in head injury. *J Neurosurg* 67:832-830, 1987.

126. Mayhall, C.G., N.H. Archer, V.A. Lamb, and et al, Ventriculostomy-related infections. A prospective epidemiologic study. *N Engl J Med* 310:553-550, 1984.

127. McQueen, J.K., D.H. Blackwood, P. Harris, R.M. Kalbag, and A.L. Johnson, Low risk of late post-traumatic seizures following severe head injury: implications for clinical trials of prophylaxis. *J.Neurol. Neurosurg. Psychiatry* 46:899-904, 1983.

128. McQueen, J.K., D.H.R. Blackwood, P. Harris, and et al, Low risk of late post-traumatic seizures following severe head injury: Implications for clinical trials of prophylaxis. *J Neurol Neurosurg Psychiatry* 46:899-904, 1983.

129. Miller, J. and J. Pickard, Intracranial volume/pressure studies in patients with head injury. *Injury* 5:265-260, 1974.

130. Miller, J.D., J.F. Butterworth, S. Gudeman, and et al, Further experience in the management of severe head injury. *J Neurosurg* 54:289-299, 1981.

131. Monro, A. *Observations on the Structure and Function of the Nervous System*, Edinburgh:Creech and Johnson, 1783.

132. Muizelaar, J.P. Cerebral blood flow measurements in the diagnosis and treatment of aneurysmal vasospasm. In: *Cerebral Vasospasm*, edited by Wilkins, R.H. New York: Raven Press, 1988, p. 63-72.

133. Muizelaar, J.P. Induced arterial hypertension in the treatment of high ICP. In: *Intracranial Pressure VII*, edited by Hoff, J.T. Berlin: Springer-Verlag, 1991,

134. Muizelaar, J.P. and D.P. Becker, Induced hypertension for the treatment of cerebral ischemia after subarachnoid hemorrhage. Direct effect on cerebral blood flow. *Surg Neurol* 25:317-325, 1986.

135. Muizelaar, J.P., H.A. Lutz, D.P. and Becker, Effect of mannitol on ICP and CBF and correlation with pressure autoregulation in severely head-injured patients. *J Neurosurg* 61:700-706, 1984.

136. Muizelaar, J.P., A. Marmarou, A.A.F. DeSalles, and et al, Cerebral blood flow and metabolism in severely head injured children. Part I: Relation with GCS, outcome, ICP and PVI. *J Neurosurg* 1991.

137. Muizelaar, J.P., E.P. Wei, H.A. Kontos, and et al, Cerebral blood flow is regulated by changes in blood pressure and in blood viscosity alike. *Stroke* 17:44-48, 1986.

138. Muizelaar, J.P., H.G. van der Poel, Z. Li, and et al, Pial arteriolar vessel diameter and CO_2 reactivity during prolonged hyperventilation in the rabbit. *J Neurosurg* 69:923-927, 1988.

139. Murphy, T.H., M. Miyamoto, A. Sastre, R.L. Schnaar, and J.T. Coyle, Glutamate toxicity in a neuronal cell line involves inhibition of cystine transport leading to oxidative stress. *Neuron.* 2:1547-1558, 1989.

140. Narayan, R.K., P.R.S. Kishore, D.P. Becker, and et al, Intracranial pressure: To monitor or not to monitor. *J Neurosurg* 56:650, 1982.

141. Nath, F. and S. Galbraith, The effect of mannitol on cerebral white matter water content. *J Neurosurg* 65:41-40, 1986.

142. Nelson, R.J., S. Perry, T.K. Hames, and J.D. Pickard, Transcranial Doppler ultrasound studies of cerebral autoregulation and subarachnoid hemorrhage in the rabbit. *J Neurosurg* 73:601-610, 1990.

143. Nelson, R.J., S. Perry, T.K. Hames, and J.D. Pickard, Transcranial Doppler ultrasound studies of cerebral autoregulation and subarachnoid hemorrhage in the rabbit. *J Neurosurg.* 73:601-610, 1990.

144. Nicholls, D.G. and T.S. Sihra, Synaptosomes possess an exocytotic pool of glutamate. *Nature* 321:772-773, 1986.

145. North, J.B. andS. Jennett, Abnormal breathing patterns associated with acute brain damage. *Arch Neurol* 31:338-344, 1974.

146. Norton, L., J. Greer, and B. Eisman, Gastric secretory response to head injury. *Arch Surg* 101:200, 1970.

147.   Obrist, W.D., T. Langfitt, J.L. Jaggi, and et al, Cerebral blood flow and metabolism in comatose patients with acute head injury: Relationship to intracranial hypertension. *J Neurosurg* 61:241-253, 1984.

148.   Olivares, L., A. Segovia, and R. Revuelta, Tube feeding and lethal aspiration in neurological patients: A review of 720 autopsy cases. *Stroke* 5:654-650, 1974.

149.   Olney, J.W., R.C. Collins, and R.S. Sloviter, Excitotoxic mechanisms of epileptic brain damage. *Adv Neurol* 44:857-877, 1986.

150.   Origitano, T.C., T.M. Wascher, O.H. Reichman, and D.E. Anderson, Sustained increased cerebral blood flow with prophylactic hypertensive hypervolemic hemodilution ("triple-H" therapy) after subarachnoid hemorrhage. *Neurosurgery*. 27:729-39; discuss, 1990.

151.   Pasqualin, A., D.G. Vollmer, J.A. Marron, T. Tsukahara, N.F. Kassell, and J.C. Torner, The effect of nicardipine on vasospasm in rabbit basilar artery after subarachnoid hemorrhage. *Neurosurgery*. 29:183-188, 1991.

152.   Pennington, J.E. Recent advances in the treatment of pneumonia in the intensive care unit. *J Hosp Infect* 11(A):295-290, 1988.

153.   Pennza, P.T. Aspiration pneumonia, necrotizing pneumonia, and lung abscess. *Emerg Med Clin North Am* 7:279-270, 1989.

154.   Pitts, E. and J. Katkis, Effect of megadose steroids on ICP in traumatic coma. In: *Intracranial Pressure IV*, edited by Shulman, K., Marmarou, A. and Miller, A. New York: Springer-Verlag, 1972, p. 638-630.

155.   Plum, F. What causes infarction in ischemic brain ? The Robert Wartenberg Lecture. *Neurology* 33:222-233, 1983.

156.   Plum, F. and J.B. Posner, Major diagnostic laboratory procedures: Electroencephalogram. In: *The Diagnosis of Stupor and Coma*, edited by Plum, F. and Posner, J.B. Philadelphia: F.A. Davis Co., 1980, p. 70-72.

157.   Pollay, M., C. Fullenwider, P.A. Roberts, and et al, Effect of mannitol and furosemide on blood-brain osmotic gradient and intracranial pressure. *J Neurosurg* 59:945-940, 1983.

158.   Przuntek, H., F. von Baumgarten, and H.G. Mertens, Treatment of vasospasm due to subarachnoid hemorrhage with calcium entry blockers. *Eur. Neurol* 25 Suppl 1:86-92, 1986.

159.   Ramsey, R.E. Electrophysiological recording in the ICU. In: *Intensive Care for Neurological Trauma and Disease*, edited by Green, B.A., Marshall, L.F. and Gallagher, T.J. New York: Academic Press, 1982, p. 177-200.

160.   Robinson, M.B. and J.T. Coyle, Glutamate and related acidic excitatory neurotransmitters: from basic science to clinical application. *FASEB. J* 1:446-455, 1987.

161.   Rodriguez, P. Gaetani, F. Marzatico, G. Benzi, L. Pacchiarini, and P. Paoletti, Effects of nicardipine on the ex vivo release of eicosanoids after experimental subarachnoid hemorrhage. *J Neurosurg* 71:903-908, 1989.

162.   Romner, B., L. Brandt, L. Berntman, L. Algotsson, B. Ljunggren, and K. Messeter, Simultaneous transcranial Doppler sonography and cerebral blood flow measurements of cerebrovascular CO_2-reactivity in patients with aneurysmal subarachnoid hemorrhage. *Br J Neurosurg* 5:31-37, 1991.

163.   Romner, B., B. Ljunggren, L. Brandt, and H. Saveland, Transcranial Doppler sonography within 12 hours after subarachnoid hemorrhage. *J Neurosurg* 70:732-736, 1989.

164.   Rosenwasser RH, D.F. Jimenez Early Aneurysm Surgery : Preliminary Results in 184 Patients. *Proceedings of the A.A.N.S.* April:1991.(Abstract)

165.   Rosenwasser, R.H. Elevated Systemic Vascular Resistance As An Indicator OF Cerebral Vasospasm After Subarachnoid Hemorrhage. *Proceedings of A.A.N.S* 1986.(Abstract)

166.   Rosenwasser, R.H., D.A. Andrews, and D.F. Jimenez, Penetrating craniocerebral trauma. *Surgical Clinics of North America* 71(2):304-316, 1991.

167.   Rosenwasser, R.H., W.A. Buchheit, and R.C. Truex, Jr. Management of subarachnoid hemorrhage. *Pa. Med.* 87:72, 74, 76, 1984.

168.   Rosenwasser, R.H., T.E. Delgado, W.A. Buchheit, and M.H. Freed, Control of hypertension and prophylaxis against vasospasm in cases of subarachnoid hemorrhage: a preliminary report. *Neurosurgery.* 12:658-661, 1983.

169.   Rosenwasser, R.H., L.I. Kleiner, J.P. Krzeminski,and W.A. Buchheit, Intracranial pressure monitoring in the posterior fossa: a preliminary report. *J.Neurosurg.* 71:503-505, 1989.

170.   Rosenwasser, R.H. and J. Winer, Acute barbiturate therapy in head injury: A systematic approach. *A.A.N.S . Meeting* 1990.

171. Rosenwasser, R.H., W. Young, Complications of hemodynamic monitoring in subarachnoid hemorrhage. *Proceedings of the A.A.N.S.-5/92* 1992.(Abstract)

172. Rosner, M.J. and D.P. Becker, Experimental brain injury: Successful therapy with the weak base, tromethamine with an overview of CNS acidosis. *J Neurosurg* 60:961-960, 1984.

173. Rosner, M.J. and I.B. Coley, Cerebral perfusion pressure, intracranial pressure, and head elevation. *J Neurosurg* 60:636-630, 1986.

174. Rosner, M.J., K.G. Elias, and I. Coley, Prospective, randomized trial of THAM therapy in severe brain injury: Preliminary results. In: *Intracranial Pressure VII*, edited by Hoff, J.T. and Betz, A.L. Berlin: Springer-Verlag, 1989, p. 611-610.

175. Rowlands, B.J., N.S. Litofsky, and H.H. Kaufman, Metabolic physiology, pathophysiology and management. In: *Neurosurgical Critical Care*, edited by Mirth, F.P. and Ratcheson, R.A. Baltimore: Williams & Wilkins, 1987, p. 81-108.

176. Rumpl, E., M. Prugger, G. Gerstenbrand, and et al, Central somatosensory conduction time and acoustic brainstem transmission time in post-traumatic coma. *J Clin Neurophysiol* 5:237-260, 1988.

177. Sadick, N.S. Sclerotherapy of varicose and telangiectatic leg veins. Minimal sclerosant concentration of hypertonic saline and its relationship to vessel diameter. *J. Dermatol. Surg. Oncol.* 17:65-70, 1991.

178. Sahlin, C., J. Brismar, T. Delgado, C. Owman, L.G. Salford, and N.A. Svendgaard, Cerebrovascular and metabolic changes during the delayed vasospasm following experimental subarachnoid hemorrhage in baboons, and treatment with a calcium antagonist. *Brain Res.* 403:313-332, 1987.

179. Sahs, A.L., H. Nishioka, J.C. Torner, C.J. Graf, N.F. Kassell, and L.C. Goettler, Cooperative study of intracranial aneurysms and subarachnoid hemorrhage: a long-term prognostic study. I. Introduction. *Arch Neurol* 41:1140-1141, 1984.

180. Sande, J.J. and J.J. Van der Velkamp, Head injury and coagulation disorders. *J Neurosurg* 94:357-350, 1978.

181. Saul, T.G. and T.B. Ducker, Effects of intracranial pressure monitoring and aggressive treatment on mortality in severe head injury. *J Neurosurg* 56:498-490, 1982.

182. Saul, T.G., T.B. Ducker, M. Saleman, and et al, Steroids in severe head injury. A prospective, randomized clinical trial. *J Neurosurg* 54:596-590, 1981.

183. Schievink, W.I., D.J. van der Werf, L.M. Hageman, and J.J. Dreissen, Referral pattern of patients with aneurysmal subarachnoid hemorrhage. *Surg Neurol* 29:367-371, 1988.

184. Schmall, L.M., W.W. Muir, J.T. and Robertson, Haemodynamic effects of small volume hypertonic saline in experimentally induced hemorrhagic shock. *Equine. Vet.J* . 22:273-277, 1990.

185. Schmall, L.M., W.W. Muir, J.T. and Robertson, Hematological, serum electrolyte and blood gas effects of small volume hypertonic saline in experimentally induced hemorrhagic shock. *Equine. Vet.J* . 22:278-283, 1990.

186. Schmidt, J.F., G. Waldemar, S. Vorstrup, A.R. Andersen, F. Gjerris, and O.B. Paulson, Computerized analysis of cerebral blood flow autoregulation in humans: validation of a method for pharmacologic studies. *J. Cardiovasc. Pharmacol.* 15:983-988, 1990.

187. Schor, N.F. Inactivation of mammalian brain glutamine synthetase by oxygen radicals. *Brain Res.* 456:17-21, 1988.

188. Seiler, R.W., P. Grolimund, H.R. and Zurbruegg, Evaluation of the calcium-antagonist nimodipine for the prevention of vasospasm after aneurysmal subarachnoid hemorrhage. A prospective transcranial Doppler ultrasound study. *Acta Neurochir* 85:7-16, 1987.

189. Seiler, R.W., H.J. Reulen, P. Huber, P. Grolimund, U. Ebeling, U. and H.J. Steiger, Outcome of aneurysmal subarachnoid hemorrhage in a hospital population: a prospective study including early operation, intravenous nimodipine, and transcranial Doppler ultrasound. *Neurosurgery.* 23:598-604, 1988.

190. Seisjo, B.K. Cell damage in the brain: A speculative synthesis. *J Cereb Blood Flow Metab* 1:155-185, 1981.

191. Seisjo, B.K. and T. Wieloch, Brain injury: Neurochemical agents. In: *Central Nervous System Trauma: Status Report*, edited by Becker, D.P. and Povlishock, J.T. Bethesda: National Institute of Neurological and Communicative Disorders and Stroke, 1985, p. 513-532.

192. Seitz, W., J. Kaukemuller, and G. Frank, [Complications caused by a Swan-Ganz catheter. An inadvertent entrapment in the right atrium during cardiac surgery]. *Anesthesist.* 38:259-261, 1989.

193. Shackford, S.R. Hypertonic saline for postoperative fluid therapy: salient features. *J. Trauma.* 29:894, 1989.

194. Shackford, S.R. Hypertonic saline and dextran for intraoperative fluid therapy: more for less. *Crit. Care. Med.* 20:160-162, 1992.

195. Shackford, S.R., J.W. Davis, P. Hollingsworth-Fridlund, and et al, Venous thromboembolism in patients with major trauma. *Am J Surg* 159:365-360, 1990.

196. Shackford, S.R., D.A. Fortlage, R.M. Peters, P. Hollingsworth-Fridlund, and M.J. Sise, Serum osmolar and electrolyte changes associated with large infusions of hypertonic sodium lactate for intravascular volume expansion of patients undergoing aortic reconstruction. *Surg. Gynecol. Obstet.* 164:127-136, 1987.

197. Shapiro, H.M. and L.F. Marshall, Intracranial pressure responses to PEEP in head injured patients. *J Trauma* 18:254-256, 1978.

198. Sharborough, F.W. and T.M. Sundt, Jr., Electroencephalography. In: *Neurological Surgery*, edited by Youmans, J.R. Philadelphia: W.B. Saunders Company, 1982, p. 195-230.

199. Shenaq, S.A., G.P. Noon, J.L. Zamora, D.H. Morrow, and D. Hoover, Unusual complication of Swan-Ganz catheter requiring mediastinotomy. *South. Med. J.* 77:1339, 1984.

200. Shimm, D.S. and L. Rigsby, Ventricular tachycardia associated with removal of a Swan-Ganz catheter. *Postgrad. Med.* 67:291, 294, 1980.

201. Shimoda, M., S. Yamada, I. Yamamoto, R. Tsugane, and O. Sato, Time course of CSF lactate level in subarachnoid hemorrhage. Correlation with clinical grading and prognosis. *Acta Neurochir* 99:127-134, 1989.

202. Sieber, F.E., R.C. Koehler, S.A. Derrer, C.D. Saudek, and R.J. Traystman, Hypoglycemia and cerebral autoregulation in anesthetized dogs. *Am. J. Physiol.* 258:H1714-H1721, 1990.

203. Sinha, R.P., T.B. Ducker, and P.L. Perot, Arterial oxygenation. Findings and its significance in central nervous system trauma patients. *JAMA* 224:1258-1260, 1973.

204. Slung, H.B. and K.S. Scher, Complications of the Swan-Ganz catheter. *World. J. Surg.* 8:76-81, 1984.

205. Sly, P.D. and C.J. Lanteri, Site of action of hypertonic saline in the canine lung. *J. Appl. Physiol.* 71:1315-1321, 1991.

206.   Smith, R.W. and J.F. Alksne,   Infections complicating the use of external ventriculostomy. *J Neurosurg* 44:567-560, 1976.

207.   Soliman, M.H., H. Ragab, and K. Waxman, Survival after hypertonic saline resuscitation from hemorrhage. *Am. Surg.* 56:749-751, 1990.

208.   Solomon, R.A. and M.E. Fink, Current strategies for the management of aneurysmal subarachnoid hemorrhage. *Arch Neurol* 44:769-774, 1987.

209.   Solomon, R.A., M.E. Fink, and L. Lennihan,   Early aneurysm surgery and prophylactic hypervolemic hypertensive therapy for the treatment of aneurysmal subarachnoid hemorrhage. *Neurosurgery.* 23:699-704, 1988.

210.   Spencer, S.S. Surgical options for uncontrolled epilepsy. *Neurol. Clin.* 4:669-695, 1986.

211.   Stange, K., M. Lagerkranser,   and A. Sollevi,   Effect of adenosine-induced hypotension on the cerebral autoregulation in the anesthetized pig. *Acta Anesthesiol. Scand.* 33:450-457, 1989.

212.   Stange, K., M. Lagerkranser, and A. Sollevi, Nitroprusside-induced hypotension and cerebrovascular autoregulation in the anesthetized pig. *Anesth. Analg.* 73:745-752, 1991.

213.   Steinke, D.E., B.K.A. Weir, J.M. Findlay, and et al,   A trial of the 21-aminosteroid U74006F in a primate model of chronic cerebral vasospasm. *Neurosurg.* 24:179-170, 1989.

214.   Stevens, M.K., T.L. Yaksh, R.B. Hansen, and R.E. Anderson, Effect of preischemia cyclooxygenase inhibition by zomepirac sodium on reflow, cerebral autoregulation, and EEG recovery in the cat after global ischemia. *J. Cereb. Blood. Flow. Metab,* 6:691-702, 1986.

215.   Stone, J.L., R.F. Ghaly, and J.R. Hughes, Electroencephalography in acute head injury. *J Clin Neurophysiol* 5:125-133, 1988.

216.   Sugi, T., M. Fujishima, and T. Omae, Lactate and pyruvate concentrations, and acid-base balance of cerebrospinal fluid in experimentally induced intracerebral and subarachnoid hemorrhage in dogs. *Stroke.* 6:715-719, 1975.

217.   Svendgaard, N.A., J. Brismar, T. Delgado, et al. Late cerebral arterial spasm: the cerebrovascular response to hypercapnia, induced hypertension and the effect of nimodipine on blood flow autoregulation in experimental subarachnoid hemorrhage in primates. *Gen. Pharmacol.* 14:167-172, 1983.

218.   Symon, L. Flow thresholds in brain ischemia and the effects of drugs. *Br J Anesth* 57:34-43, 1985.

219.   Synek, V.M. Prognostically important EEG coma patterns in diffuse anoxic and traumatic encephalopathies in adults. *J Clin Neurophysiol* 5:161-174, 1988.

220.   Takeuchi, H., Y. Handa, H. Kobayashi, H. Kawano, and M. Hayashi, Impairment of cerebral autoregulation during the development of chronic cerebral vasospasm after subarachnoid hemorrhage in primates. *Neurosurgery.* 28:41-48, 1991.

221.   Tanaka, K., F. Gotoh, F. Muramatsu, et al. Effect of nimodipine, a calcium antagonist, on cerebral vasospasm after subarachnoid hemorrhage in cats. *Arzneimittelforschung.* 32:1529-1534, 1982.

222.   Temkin, N.R., S.S. Dikmen, A.J. Wilensky, J. Keihm, S. Chabal, and H.R. Winn, A randomized, double-blind study of phenytoin for the prevention of post-traumatic seizures. *N. Engl. J. Med.* 323:497-502, 1990.

223.   Theodore, J. and E.D. Robin, Pathogenesis of neurogenic pulmonary edema. *Lancet* 2:749-751, 1975.

224.   Theodore, J. and E.D. Robin, Speculations on neurogenic pulmonary edema. *Am Rev Resp Dis* 113:405-411, 1976.

225.   Todd, M.M., S.M. Toutant, H.M. and Shapiro, The effects of high-frequency positive pressure ventilation on intracranial pressure and brain surface movement in cats. *Anesthesiology* 54:496-504, 1981.

226.   Toyota, A. and Y. Nishizawa, [Cerebral vasospasm after subarachnoid hemorrhage, and inhibitory effect of nicardipine investigated by means of transcranial Doppler ultrasonography]. *No. Shinkei. Geka.* 19:1143-1150, 1991.

227.   Tsutsume, H., K. Ide, T. Mizutani, and et al, The relationship between intracranial pressure, cerebral perfusion pressure, and outcome in head-injured patients: The critical level of cerebral perfusion pressure. In: *Intracranial Pressure VI*, edited by Miller, J., Teasdale, G., Rowan, J. and et al, Berlin: Springer-Verlag, 1986, p. 661-660.

228.   Turner, D.M., N.F. Kassell, T. Sasaki, Y.G. Comair, D.O. Beck, and S.L. Klein, Cerebral and systemic vascular effects of naloxone in pentobarbital-anesthetized normal dogs. *Neurosurgery.* 14:276-282, 1984.

229. Tuyman, D., A.B. Young, J.A. Norton, and et al, High protein enteral feedings: A means of achieving positive nitrogen balance in head injured patients. *JPEN* 9:679-684, 1985.

230. Uzell, B.P., W.D. Obrist, C.A. Dolinskas, and et al, Relationship of acute CBF and ICP findings to neuropsychological outcome in severe head injury. *J Neurosurg* 65:630-635, 1986.

231. Uziel, A. and J. Benezech, Auditory brain-stem responses in comatose patients. Relationships with brain-stem reflexes and levels of coma. *Electroencephalogr Clin Neurophysiol* 45:515-524, 1978.

232. Verlooy, J., L. Heytens, E. Van den Brande, and P. Selosse, Transcranial Doppler sonography in subarachnoid hemorrhage. *Acta Neurol Belg.* 89:346-351, 1989.

233. Volpin, L., D. Curri, M. Zanusso, P. Cervellini, A. and Benedetti, Post-SAH vasospasm in patients treated with oral nimodipine. *Riv. Eur. Sci. Med Farmacol.* 9:179-183, 1987.

234. Ward, J., D. Becker, J. Miller, and et al, Failure of prophylactic barbiturate coma in the treatment of severe head injury. *J Neurosurg* 62:383-380, 1985.

235. Ward, J.D., S. Choi, A. Marmarou, and et al, Effect of prophylactic hyperventilation on outcome in patients with severe head injury. In: *Intracranial Pressure VII*, edited by Hoff, J.T. and Betz, A.L. Berlin: Springer-Verlag, 1989, p. 630.

236. White, P.F., R.M. Schlobohm, L.H. Pitts, and et al, A randomized study of drugs for preventing increases in intracranial pressure during endotracheal suctioning. *Anesthesiology* 57:242-240, 1982.

237. Wilkinson, H.A. and S.R. Rosenfeld, Furosemide and mannitol in the treatment of experimental intracranial hypertension. *Neurosurg.* 12:405-400, 1983.

238. Winer, J.W., R.H. Rosenwasser, and F.Jimenez, Electroencephalographic activity and serum and cerebrospinal fluid pentobarbital levels in determining the therapeutic end point during barbiturate coma. *Neurosurgery.* 29:739-41; discuss, 1991.

239. Winn, H.R., S. Morii, R.M. and Berne, The role of adenosine in autoregulation of cerebral blood flow. *Ann. Biomed. Eng.* 13:321-328, 1985.

240. Wronski, J., R. Abraszko, W. Berny, J. and Mierzwa, Clinical experiences with nimodipine treatment in patients after SAH and aneurysm surgery. *Zentralbl. Neurochir* 51:21-23, 1990.

241. Yano, M., H. Nishiyama, H. Yokota, and et al, Effect of lidocaine on ICP response to endotracheal suctioning. *Anesthesiology* 64:651-650, 1986.

242. Young, B., R.P. Rapp, J.A. Norton, D. Haack, J.W. and Walsh, Failure of prophylactically administered phenytoin to prevent post-traumatic seizures in children. *Childs. Brain* 10:185-192, 1983.

243. Zornow, M.H., M.S. Scheller, S.R. and Shackford, Effect of a hypertonic lactated Ringer's solution on intracranial pressure and cerebral water content in a model of traumatic brain injury. *J. Trauma.* 29:484-488, 1989.

244. Zuccarello, M., J.T. Marsch, G. Schmitt, J. Woodward, J. and D.K. Anderson, Effect of the 21-aminosteroid U-74006F on cerebral vasospasm following subarachnoid hemorrhage. *J. Neurosurg.* 71:98-104, 1989.

245. van der Poel, H. Cerebral vasoconstriction is not maintained with prolonged hyperventilation. In: *Intracranial Pressure VII*, edited by Hoff, J.T. and Betz, A.L. Berlin: Springer-Verlag, 1989,

8

MORPHOLOGIC ASPECTS OF CEREBRAL ISCHEMIA

Ehud Lavi, M.D.
Assistant Professor, Division of Neuropathology
Department of Pathology and Laboratory Medicine
University of Pennsylvania School of Medicine, Philadelphia PA 19104-6079

Dara G. Jamieson, M.D.[*]
Assistant Professor, Department of Neurology
Temple University School of Medicine. Philadelphia PA 19140

TABLE OF CONTENTS

[**] Current address: Department of Neurology, Pennsylvania Hospital, 8th and Spruce Streets, Philadelphia, PA   19107

IV. Vascular pathology in cerebral ischemia
    A. Atherosclerotic disease
    B. Hypertensive cerebrovascular disease
    C. Fibromuscular dysplasia
    D. Aortic arch syndrome
    E. Endarteritis obliterans (syphilis, TB meningitis,
       chronic pyogenic meningitis)
    F. Polyarteritis nodosa
    G. Giant cell (temporal) arteritis
    H. Wegener's granulomatosis
    I.   Systemic lupus erythematosus
    J.   Thrombotic microangiopathy
    K. Granulomatous angiitis
    L. Cerebral amyloid angiopathy

Oxygen and glucose are essential for normal brain function. The brain is exquisitely susceptible to their deprivation and irreversible changes occur within minutes. The morphological changes are essentially the same whether the deprivation is of oxygen, glucose or blood flow. When only one vessel is affected the tissue damage is localized to the territory supplied by the affected vessel in the form of cerebral infarction. When the anoxic-ischemic damage is diffuse and affecting the whole brain in conditions such as severe hypotension, cardiac arrest, severe hypoglycemia, or carbon monoxide poisoning, there are certain stereotypic morphological manifestations which result from selective vulnerability to anoxia of certain cells and specific regions in the brain [1].

I. STRUCTURAL CHANGES RESULTING FROM HYPOXIA AT THE CELLULAR LEVEL.

A. ALTERATIONS IN NEURONS.

The earliest stage of the ischemic cell process is microvacuolization of the neuronal perikaria [2]. The vacuoles represent swollen mitochondria and dilatations of the rough endoplasmic reticulum or other cytoplasmic organelles [3]. This stage may begin as early as 5-15 minutes post ischemic-anoxic insult and can be demonstrated only in experimental animals. In human the autolytic changes masquerade this phenomenon. The next stage, ischemic cell change, develops gradually after the vacuolization stage. The neurons become shrunken, with hypereosinophilic staining cytoplasm, finely dispersed Nissl substance, and shrunken, triangular, darkly stained nuclei. At a later stage, dark incrustations appear on the surface of neuronal perikaria and dendrites. These are found in experimental monkeys as early as 90 minutes and may persist for 48 hours. Electron microscopy has shown incrustations to be electron-dense profiles of neuronal cytoplasm, projecting from the cell surface which is indented and distorted by clear swollen astrocytic processes. Finally, homogenizing cell change appears after a few hours of ischemia, and may persist for 10 days or more. It is characterized by a homogeneous, eosinophilic cytoplasm with no distinctive organelles and Nissl substance, and a darkly stained granular, triangular or fragmented nucleus [4], [5], [6]. The affected neurons eventually disappear.

B. GLIAL AND MESODERMAL REACTION TO ISCHEMIA.

Glial and mesodermal reaction to ischemia is usually proportional to the size of the tissue involved and the degree and duration of ischemia. When a portion of brain parenchyma undergoes complete infarction the tissue in the center will be completely destroyed and eventually become cystic. The gliomesodermal reaction in that case will be restricted to the periphery of the infarcted area. However, in less severe ischemic damage, the affected area will be replaced by a gliomesodermal "scar". This consists of proliferating reactive astrocytes producing a network of astrocytic processes. In addition, collagen and reticulin fibers and proliferating capillaries derived from mesodermal sources participate in the formation of the scar. Another glial cell participating in the reactive process is the microglia. These become rod-shaped and proliferate in reaction to ischemia (or any other pathologic processes). After 2-3 days following ischemic insult, microglial cells may show fine lipid droplets in their cytoplasm and divisions by mitoses may be seen. Later microglia develop into typical lipid-laden macrophages. The lipid-containing macrophages do not migrate actively from the site of the damage and may persist for months. Their pattern of distribution may mirror the original destruction of the tissue.

II. ISCHEMIC HYPOXIA- GLOBAL.

This type of ischemic damage is best exemplified by generalized reduction in cerebral blood flow as in the case of severe acute hypotension or in patients who survive a cardiopulmonary arrest. In global ischemia regions and different cells in the brain have different thresholds to ischemia and selective vulnerability may be expressed in stereotypical patterns of damage [1]. However, there is also variability in presentation. The vulnerability pattern also changes with age so that the ischemic lesions of the neonatal brain are different from those of adult brain.

A. SELECTIVE CELLULAR VULNERABILITY.

Neurons are the most susceptible cell in the CNS to ischemia. Oligodendrocytes, astrocytes and microglia are less susceptible. The most resistant cells to hypoxia in the CNS are the endothelial cells [1].

B. SELECTIVELY REGIONAL VULNERABILITY.

1. Selective vulnerable locations in the adult brain.
Selective regional vulnerability of the brain to ischemia has been described in both experimental models and in humans [7], [8], [9], [10], [11], [12]. In the neocortex, the parietal and occipital lobes are more susceptible to ischemic changes than the frontal and temporal cortex. The depths of the sulci are more susceptible than the crests of the gyri (the reverse is seen in contusions). The third and fifth cortical layers are more susceptible to ischemia than the other layers. This is the reason for the appearance of laminar or pseudolaminar necrosis in severe cases of hypoxic brain damage. Several regions in the brain are especially vulnerable to ischemic damage and may present as focal injury in cases of hypotension or a short cardiorespiratory arrest. The most consistent region of such damage is the Sommer sector (CA1) of the hippocampus (Ammon's horn). Also vulnerable are CA3 and CA4 while CA2 is the most resistant part of the pyramidal cell layer of the hippocampus. The hippocampal dentate gyrus is also resistant to hypoxia. Other regions in the brain show selective vulnerability to hypoxic brain damage less frequently. These include the outer parts of the caudate and putamen, pallidum, anterior nuclear complex of the thalamus, basolateral amygdala, reticular zone of substantia nigra, inferior culliculi and inferior olives. In the cerebellum the Purkinje cells are the most vulnerable.

2. Selectively vulnerable locations in the neonatal brain.

Hypoxic brain damage in the fetus and newborn infant is responsible for a high proportion of the cases of cerebral palsy. The regional susceptibility in the developing brain is different than in the mature brain [13]. Periventricular leukomalacia with white matter necrosis, and neuronal destruction of basal ganglia and thalamus are common results of fetal hypoxic damage. Other areas which are more commonly involved in term infants include cortex, cerebellum and brainstem.

3. Boundary zone infarctions.

As a result of the unique anatomy of the cortical arterial supply, in hypotensive episodes and reduced cerebral blood flow, the flow is first reduced in boundary zones (also called watershed areas) which are the most distant parts of each circulation. These areas are between the circulations of the anterior and middle cerebral arteries, between the middle and posterior cerebral arteries and between the superior and posterior-inferior cerebellar arteries [14].

III. ISCHEMIC HYPOXIA- FOCAL: CEREBRAL INFARCTION

A. MACROSCOPIC CHANGES

The first macroscopic manifestations of an acute infarction of considerable size are swelling, congestion of blood vessels, and a soft consistency. Extravasation of blood can be grossly identified early following an hemorrhagic infarction. Within a few days after infarction the borders between infarcted and non infarcted tissue begin to be apparent and there is loss of demarcation between white and grey matter. The effect of edema especially in the white matter is maximal and mass effect can be identified macroscopically including midline shift and evidence of herniation. In 2-3 weeks following infarction the edema subsides, the tissue begins to have a granular soft texture with distinct borders. Later the infarcted tissue begins to be absorbed and cystic formation replaces it.

B. MICROSCOPIC CHANGES: TIME COURSE

Cerebral infarction can vary in size from a few millimeters to the entire territory of supply of a major blood vessel. Infarction is defined as the volume of tissue within which all cell bodies, blood vessels, and nerve fibers undergo necrosis as a result of a critical reduction in blood supply [1]. The histological changes follow a relatively predictable time course.

At 12-24 hours post infarction the major pathologic changes consist of congested vessels, early polymorphonuclear (PMN) cell infiltration at the periphery of the infarcted area and early degenerative changes in neurons and glia.

At 2-3 days post infarction, congestion of vessels reaches a peak, degenerative changes in neurons and glia are maximal, and PMNs infiltration is more abundant. There is the beginning of macrophage/microglia infiltration but at this point without myelin debris within the phagocytic cells.

At 5-7 days post infarction there is a peak of macrophage cell infiltration with maximal phagocytosis activity. The macrophages contain cellular debris and phagocytosed erythrocytes, and large amounts of myelin components which stain positively with special stains for myelin (e.g. Luxol Fast Blue) and lipids. There is beginning capillary proliferation and reactive astrocytosis especially at the edge of the infarcted area.

At 2-3 weeks post infarction capillary proliferation and reactive gliosis peak. The PMN cells disappear but the macrophages stay within the lesion. There is a beginning of transformation of incomplete ischemic damage into a glial scar.

At 1 year post infarction some macrophages persist within the lesion. Areas of complete infarction will be transformed into cystic cavities. There is reactive astrocytosis at the periphery of the lesion. Areas of incomplete damage are now fully transformed into a glial scar with fibrous astrocytes, dense astrocytic processes and mesenchymal elements including abundant blood vessels.

IV. VASCULAR PATHOLOGY IN CEREBRAL ISCHEMIA.

Blood vessels pathology is the primary cause of cerebrovascular disease. Although embolic phenomena constitute an estimated 50-60% of cerebral infarctions, the majority of those arise from a diseased proximal portion of the vessel. Cardiac emboli are responsible for approximately 20% of cerebral infarctions. The distinction between the various categories of vascular pathology relies on the following criteria: the nature and size of the diseased vessel, selective involvement of the vascular layers vs panvasculopathy, the presence or absence and the nature of the inflammatory infiltration (polymorphonuclear, lympho-plasmacytic, granulomatous), the presence or absence of microorganisms, and specific processes and substances (fibrinoid necrosis, cholesterol plaques, amyloid).

A. ATHEROSCLEROTIC DISEASE

Atherosclerosis is the major cause of cerebral vessel pathology and cerebral infarction. The process in arteries consists of focal thickening of the intima and deposition of lipids and fibrous tissue forming the so-called "atheromatous plaques" with various degrees of endothelial cell damage. Secondary changes in atheromatous plaques include ulceration, mural thrombus, calcification and aneurysmal dilatation. In small vessels such as arterioles the disease process is called arteriolarsclerosis. It involves the full thickness of the vessel with concentric thickening, fibrosis and hyalinization of all the layers of the vessel wall.

B. HYPERTENSIVE CEREBROVASCULAR DISEASE

The pathologic changes in cerebral blood vessels due to hypertension are two-fold. Hypertension leads to worsening of the atherosclerotic effect on vessels. There are also changes attributed to the pure effect of hypertension. These begin with hypertrophy of smooth muscle (media) in small arteries and arterioles. It eventually results in duplication of internal elastic lamina, hyalin deposition (fibrosis of media) and thickening of intima. The lumen of vessels affected by hypertensive changes begins to narrow and the vessel wall becomes fragile. These changes render the vessels prone to both thrombotic occlusion and rupture.

C. FIBROMUSCULAR DYSPLASIA

In fibromuscular dysplasia areas of fibrous and muscular thickening of the intima alternate with aneurysmal dilatation. It was first described in the renal arteries, but subsequently was found to exist in carotid and vertebral arteries as well [15], [16]. It occurs predominantly in women; it is bilateral in 75% of cases; and is associated with congenital aneurysms in 25% of cases.

D. AORTIC ARCH SYNDROME.

Aortic arch syndrome includes Takayasu disease in young oriental women as well as aortic arch conditions of various disease entities (including thromboarteritis obliterans, polyarteritis nodosa, giant cell arteritis, syphilis TB and atherosclerosis). It consists of a panarteritic process of the aortic arch and the origins of the innominate, left common carotid and left subclavian arteries. The pathologic findings include a granulomatous process with subsequent scarring of the vessel wall and thrombosis [17].

E. ENDARTERITIS OBLITERANS

Endarteritis obliterans is a general name for a pathologic entity seen in association with a variety of inflammatory, and chemical leptomeningeal processes. It is seen in chronic meningeal infections such as meningovascular syphilis and chronic TB meningitis. It can also be found as a sequela of chronic, unresolved, partially treated, pyogenic meningitis, or meningitis due to specific bacteria (e.g. pneumococcus). The same pathologic changes can also be experimentally produced in animals with intrathecal injections of a variety of chemicals. In endarteritis obliterans the intima and adventitia are affected with chronic mononuclear inflammation and fibrosis. The media usually remains normal with only occasional inflammation.

F. POLYARTERITIS NODOSA

Medium and small arteries and arterioles are involved in polyarteritis nodosa. The pathologic process is usually acute or subacute and involves the entire thickness of the vessel, thus panarteritis. The usual findings include subendothelial edema, fibrinoid necrosis of the media, destruction of internal elastic lamina, and inflammation which, unlike other pathologic entities, includes PMN and eosinophiles in addition to the mononuclear lymphocytic infiltration. When diseased vessels undergo healing the characteristic findings are fibrosis and occasional aneurysmal dilatation.

G. GIANT CELL (TEMPORAL) ARTERITIS - GCA

Giant cell arteritis is seen in patients over the age of 55 years with typically high erythrocyte sedimentation rate (ESR) and headache. Large and medium size arteries are focally and segmentally involved, mostly extracranially. The superficial temporal artery is frequently included and therefore used as a site for biopsy. Involvement of retinal, coronary, and internal carotid arteries can cause symptoms such as blindness, myocardial infarction and stroke. The systemic manifestations of the disease are called polymyalgia rheumatica and are associated with proximal muscle and joint pains. The pathologic findings consist of a subacute panarteritic inflammation. There is intimal proliferation, granulomatous formation including histiocytes, giant cells and lymphocytes. There is fragmentation of internal elastic lamina [18], [19], [20]. During healing there is fibrosis and aneurysmal formation. Typical pathologic findings, vessel and age distribution of GCA have been also described in patients with ESR under 25.

H. WEGENER'S GRANULOMATOSIS

Wegener's granulomatosis is a fatal systemic granulomatous arteritis involving the respiratory tract, kidneys and other organs. The brain is involved in 7% and the peripheral nervous system in 29% according to one series of 56 autopsies [21]. The pathological changes are similar to other granulomatous arteritis diseases [22].

I. SYSTEMIC LUPUS ERYTHEMATOSUS (SLE)

SLE is a multi-system disease of an autoimmune pathogenesis. The disease process involves pronounced B cell activation, resulting in the production of several polyspecific autoantibodies. Among the pathologic findings are systemic vasculitis and immune-complex disease (type III hypersensitivity). The brain is often involved in SLE, but the nature of the CNS manifestations is not clear. In autopsy series the main findings consist of multiple microinfarctions and microhemorrhages. There is rarely any evidence of vasculitis or inflammation [23]. Other factors which may contribute to CNS pathology in SLE are embolization from Libman-Sacks non-bacterial verrucous endocarditis and antineuronal antibodies.

J. THROMBOTIC MICROANGIOPATHY

Thrombotic microangiopathy describes a disease process associated with thrombotic manifestations affecting capillaries and small arterioles in the brain as well as in other organs. This pathologic process has been described in association with thrombotic thrombocytopenic purpura (TTP), hemolytic-uremic syndrome, disseminated intravascular coagulopathy (DIC) and as a paraneoplastic manifestation. The pathologic picture consists of occlusion of small blood vessels with eosinophilic material consisting of platelet and / or fibrin thrombi. This is associated with multiple microinfarctions restricted to grey matter structures. In the affected areas there is proliferation of capillaries and endothelial cells [24], [25].

K. GRANULOMATOUS ANGIITIS

This rare disease represents an intracerebral form of granulomatous arteritis, usually with a more severe clinical picture than giant cell arteritis. Although the pathologic findings of granulomatous inflammation in granulomatous angiitis are similar to those of giant cell arteritis this process is not restricted to elderly patients and it is usually not accompanied by elevated ESR [26], [27]. Small arteries and veins are involved. Several reports described "herpes like" [28] and varicella zoster particles in endothelial cells, others found mycoplasma in such cases.

L. CEREBRAL AMYLOID ANGIOPATHY - CAA

Amyloid in small and middle size cerebral arteries, arterioles, and less often veins is associated with numerous clinical syndromes, diseases and pathologic processes [29], [30], [31], [32]. Two types of familial cerebral amyloid angiopathy or hereditary cerebral hemorrhage with amyloidosis (HCHWA) have been described: the Icelandic type (HCHWA-I), and the Dutch type (HCHWA-D) [33]. Both are autosomal-dominant. A non familial cerebral amyloid angiopathy is now considered to be the main cause of spontaneous cerebral hemorrhage in the non hypertensive elderly but it can also cause cerebral microinfarctions with various clinical manifestations including dementia. Other diseases associated with cerebral amyloidosis including amyloidosis of cerebral blood vessels are: Alzheimer's disease, Down's syndrome, leukoencephalopathy, spongiform encephalopathies caused by prions, and various conditions of "secondary amyloidosis" including various forms of vasculitis.

Amyloid deposition has a predilection for temporal and occipital regions but is found rarely in the cerebellum and deep grey matter and never in the brainstem. The nature and the chemical composition of the amyloid varies in different diseases but the histologic and ultrastructural characteristics are similar. They all have beta-pleated, periodically twisted, 7-10 micron diameter fibrils which appear on H&E as amorphous eosinophilic deposition in the media and adventitia of blood vessels. It produces the "double barrel" appearance of the lumen and is often associated with fibrinoid necrosis of the vessel, and segmental dilatation with microaneurysmal formation. It can be detected with special stains for amyloid such as congo red which gives "apple green" birefringence under polarized light.

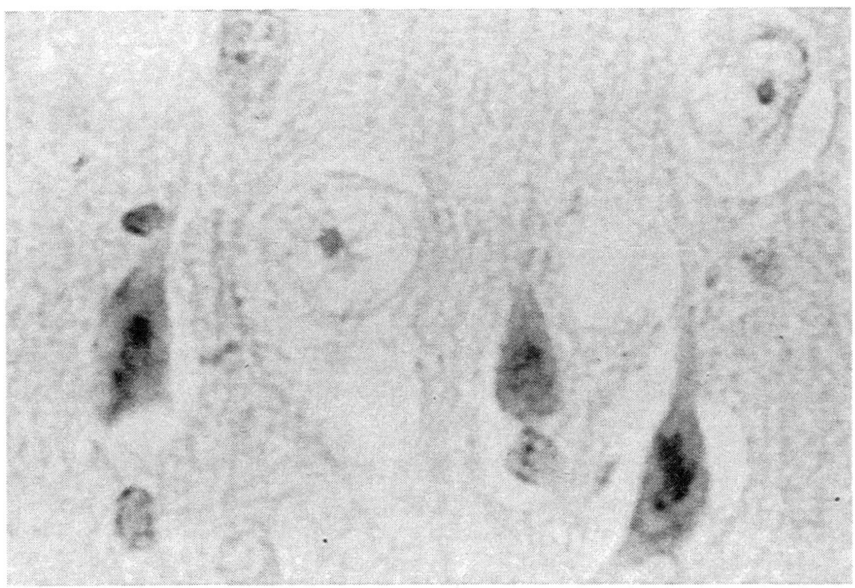

Figure 1. Ischemic cell changes in cortical neurons showing darkly stained shrunken nuclei of hypoxic neurons next to unaffected neurons. (H&E x400).

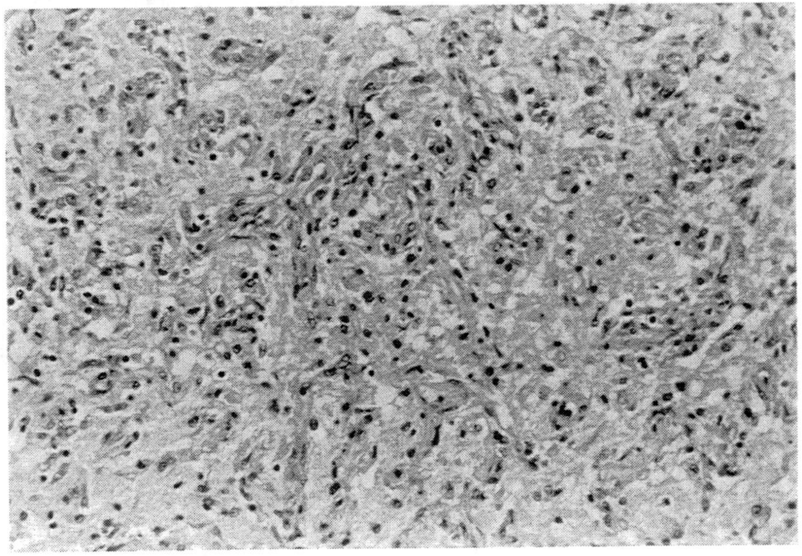

Figure 2. Extensive gliovascular reaction at the periphery of an old infarction. (H&E x200).

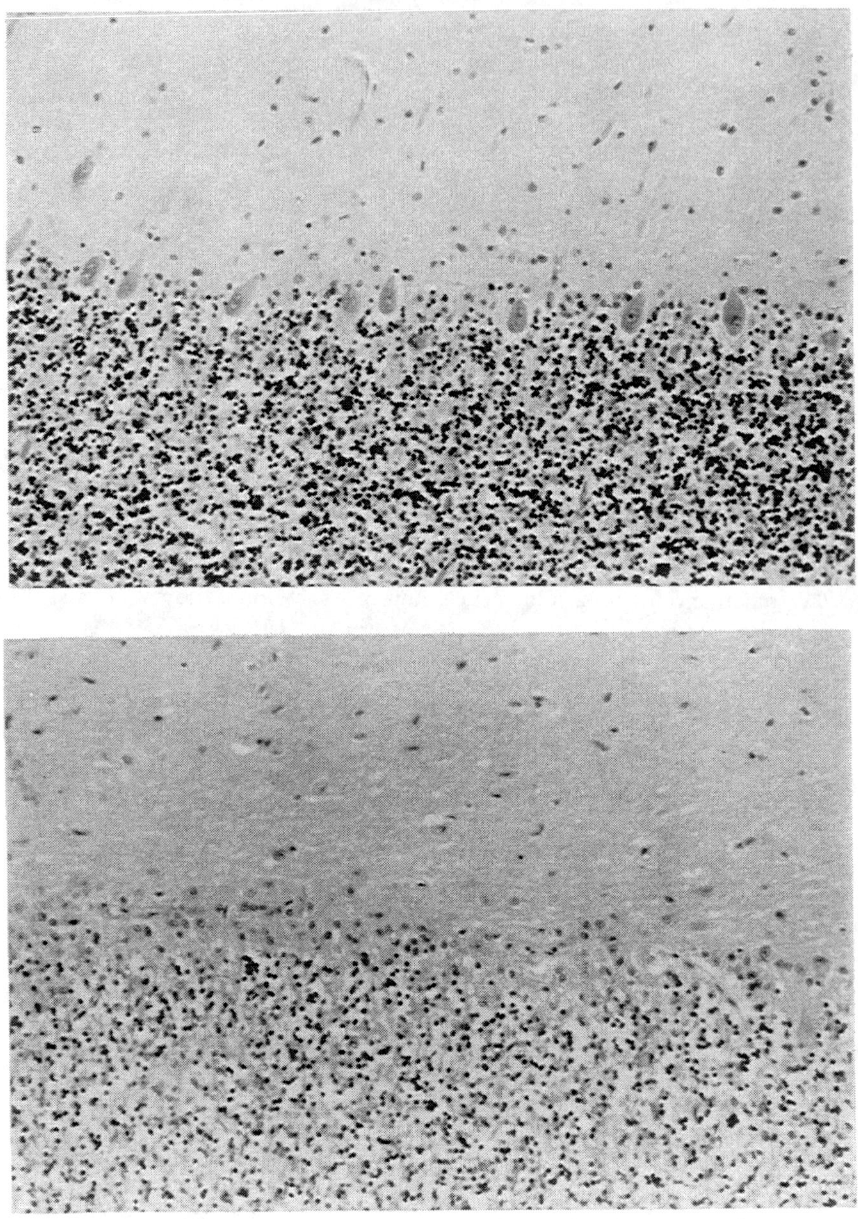

Figure 3. Selective cellular vulnerability of cerebellar Purkinje cells to global anoxia. A. Normal cerebellum. B. Loss of Purkinje cells and reactive Bergmann gliosis following cardiac arrest. (H&E x200).

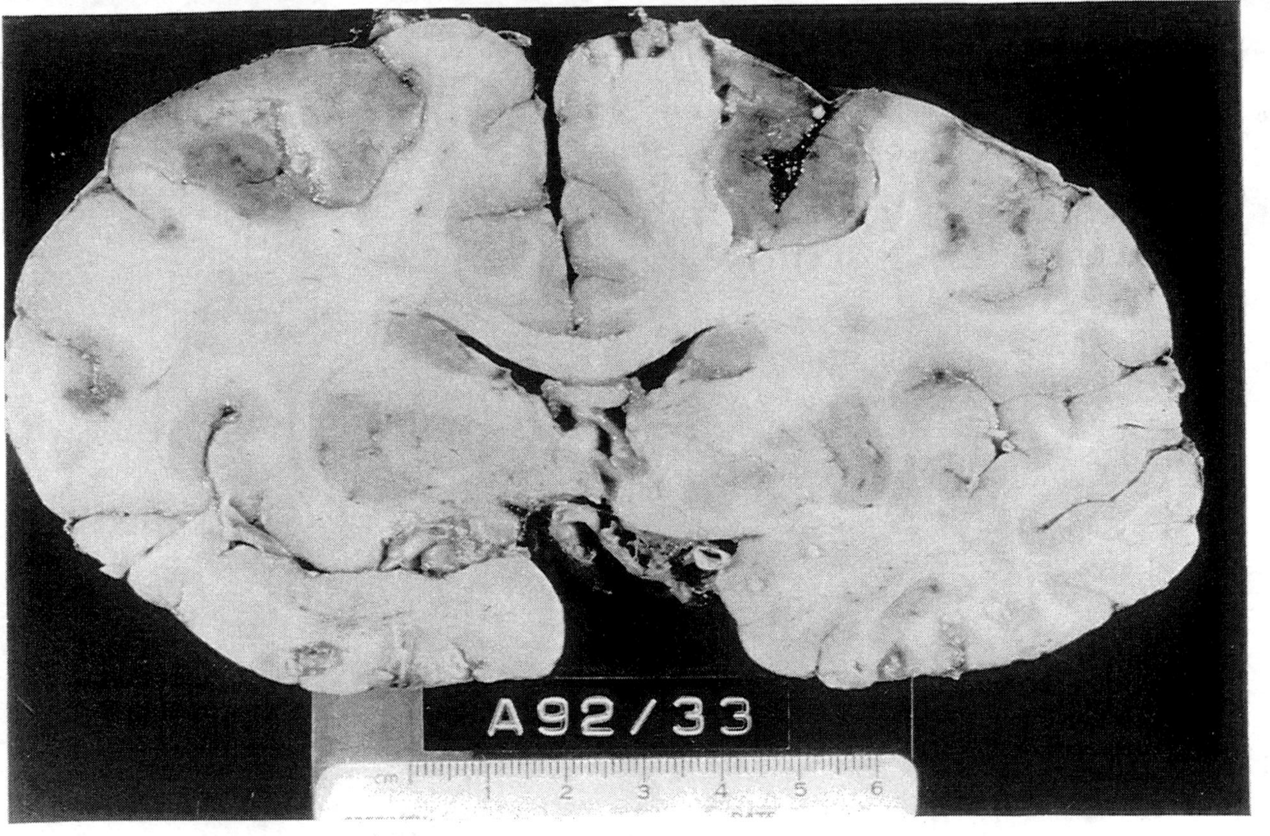

Figure 4. Coronal section of a brain showing diffuse anoxic damage most pronounced as boundary zone infarctions in the middle cerebral-anterior cerebral arteries "watershed zone" bilaterally.

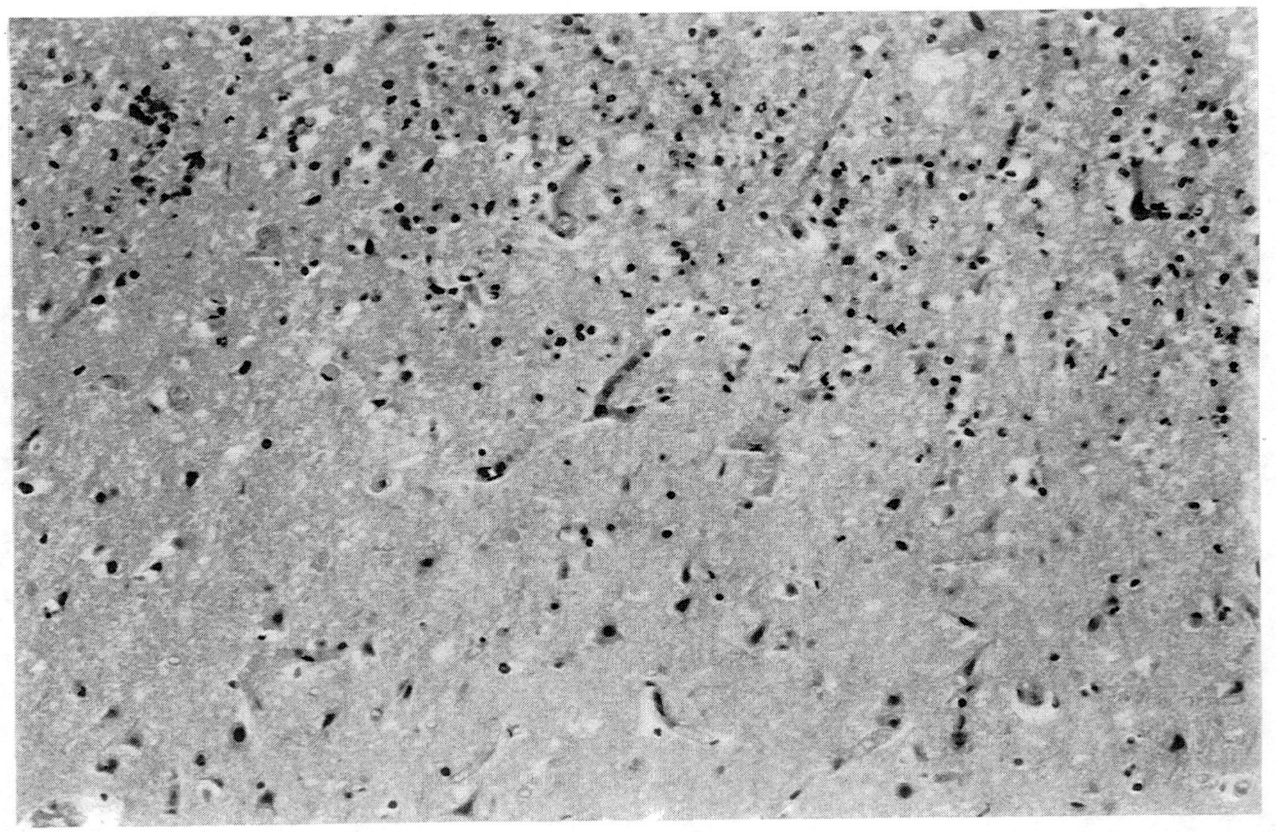

Figure 5A. Recent (24 hours) infarction showing polymorphonuclear leucocytes infiltration into the necrotic parenchyma. Note anoxic changes in neurons. (H&E x200).

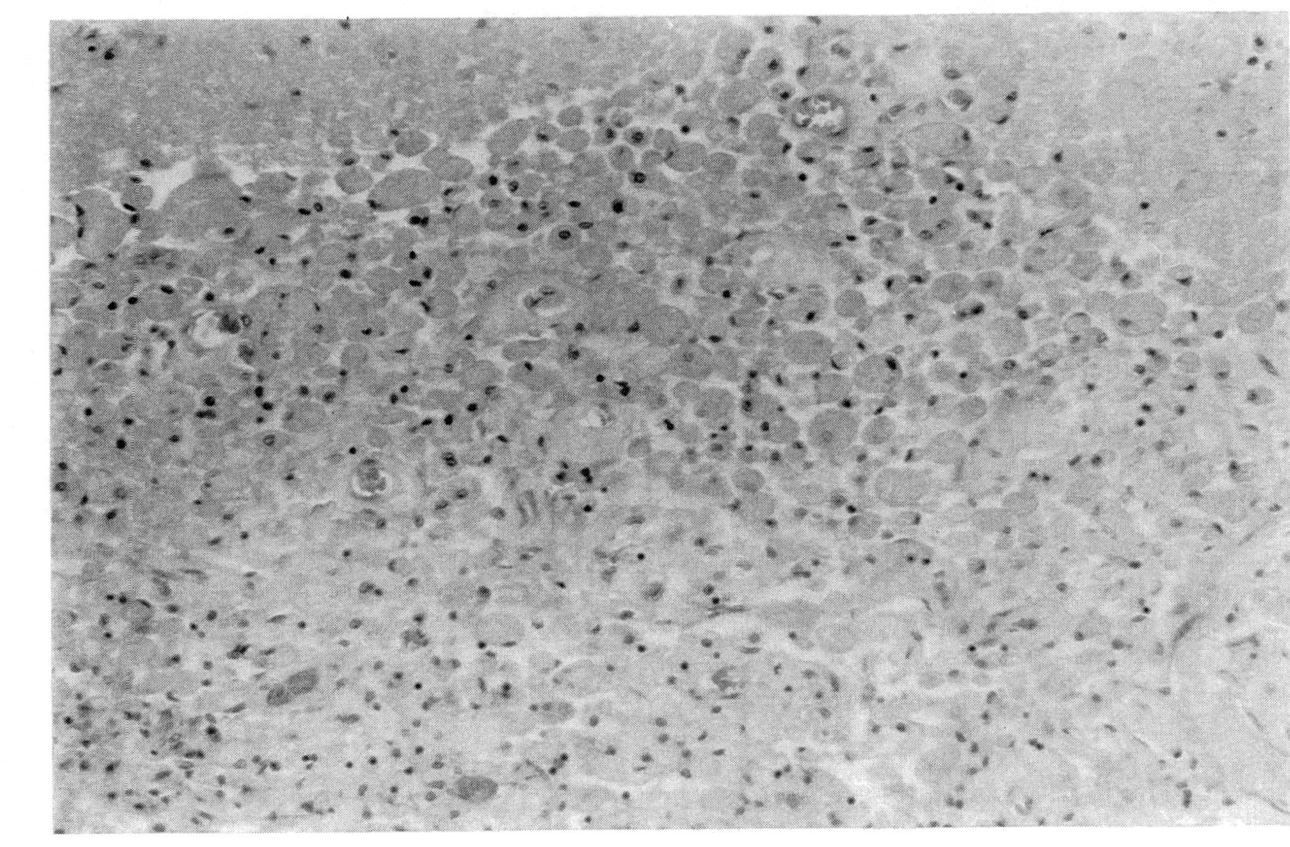

Figure 5B. Five day old cerebral infarction showing replacement of the tissue by a sea of macrophages. (H&E x200).

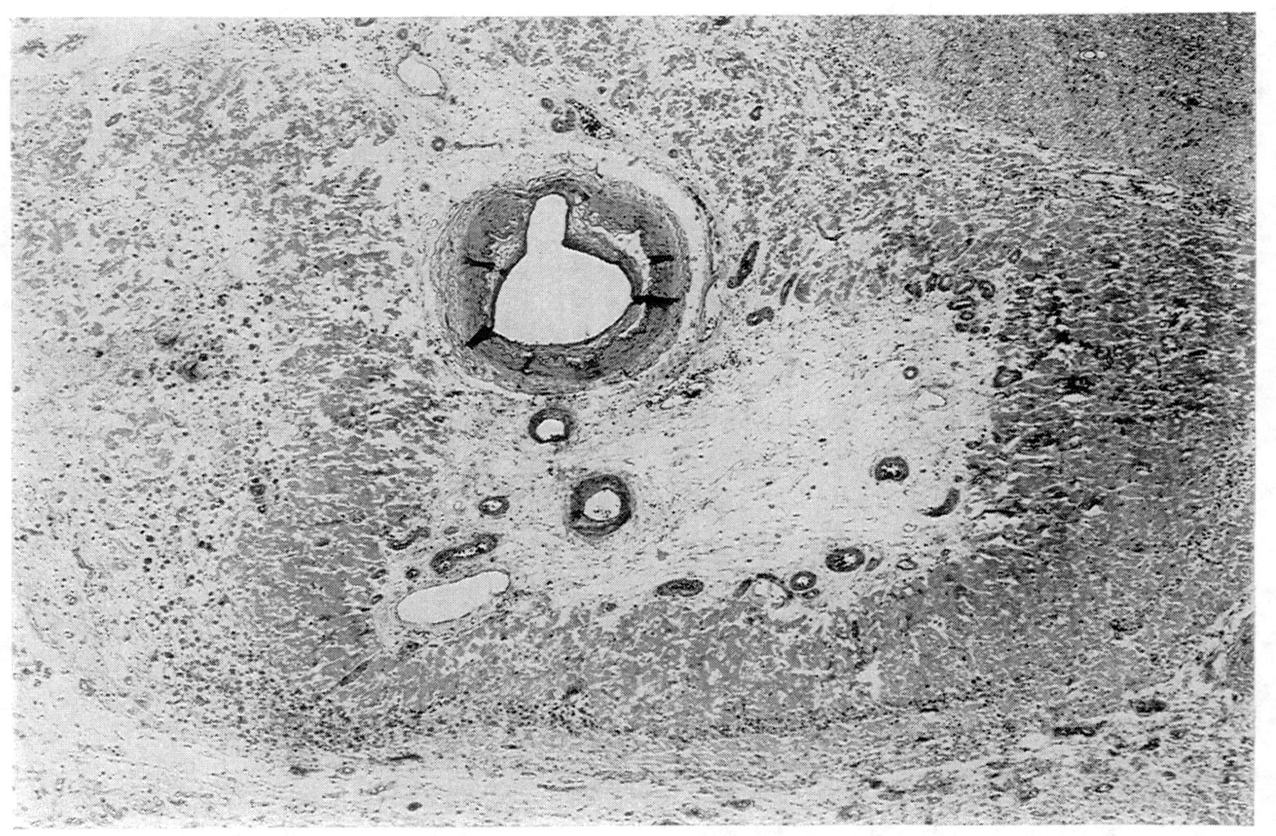

Figure 5C. Several months old infarction showing central cyst formation and of macrophage infiltration of the periphery. Note the atherosclerotic changes in a small artery. (H&E x40).

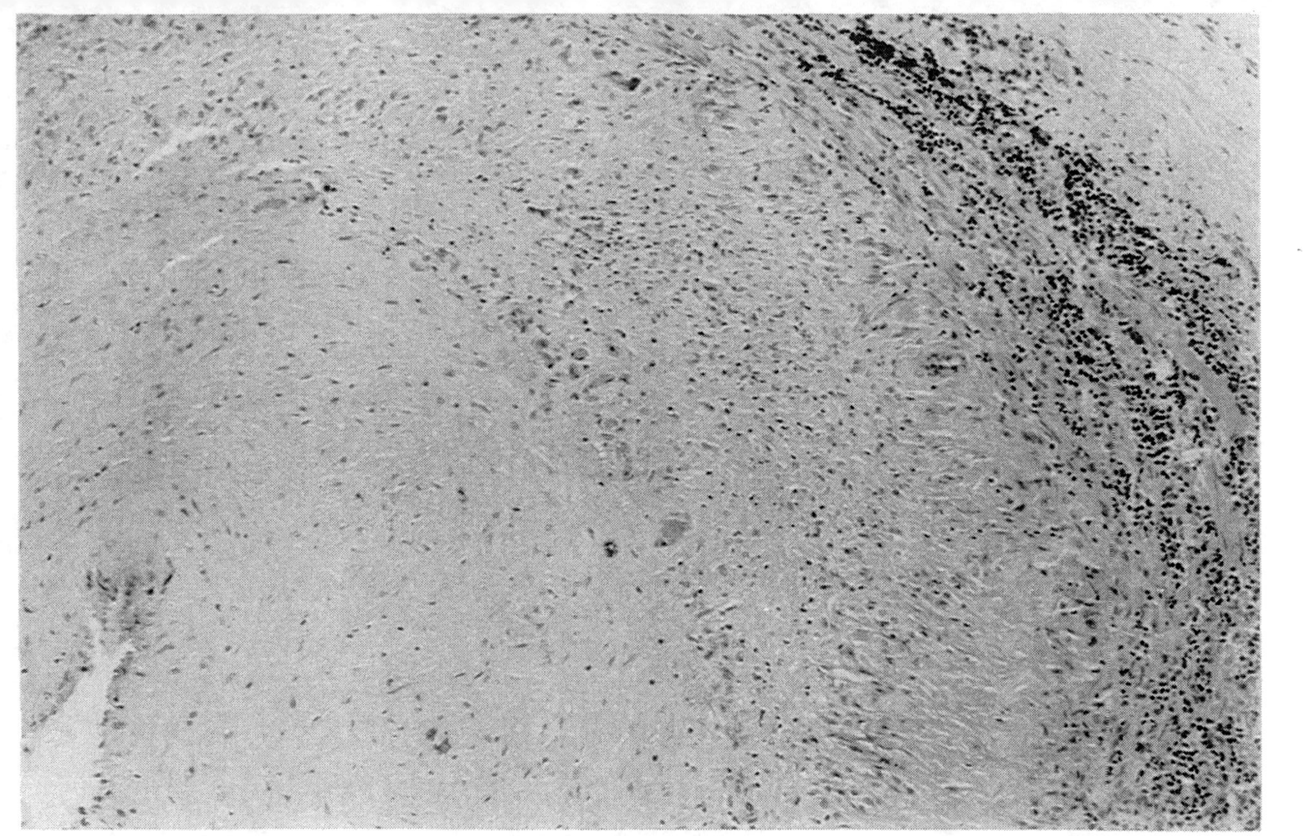

Figure 6A. Giant cell (temporal) arteritis in a section from a superficial temporal artery. Note inflammatory infiltration in the vessel wall. (H&E x40)

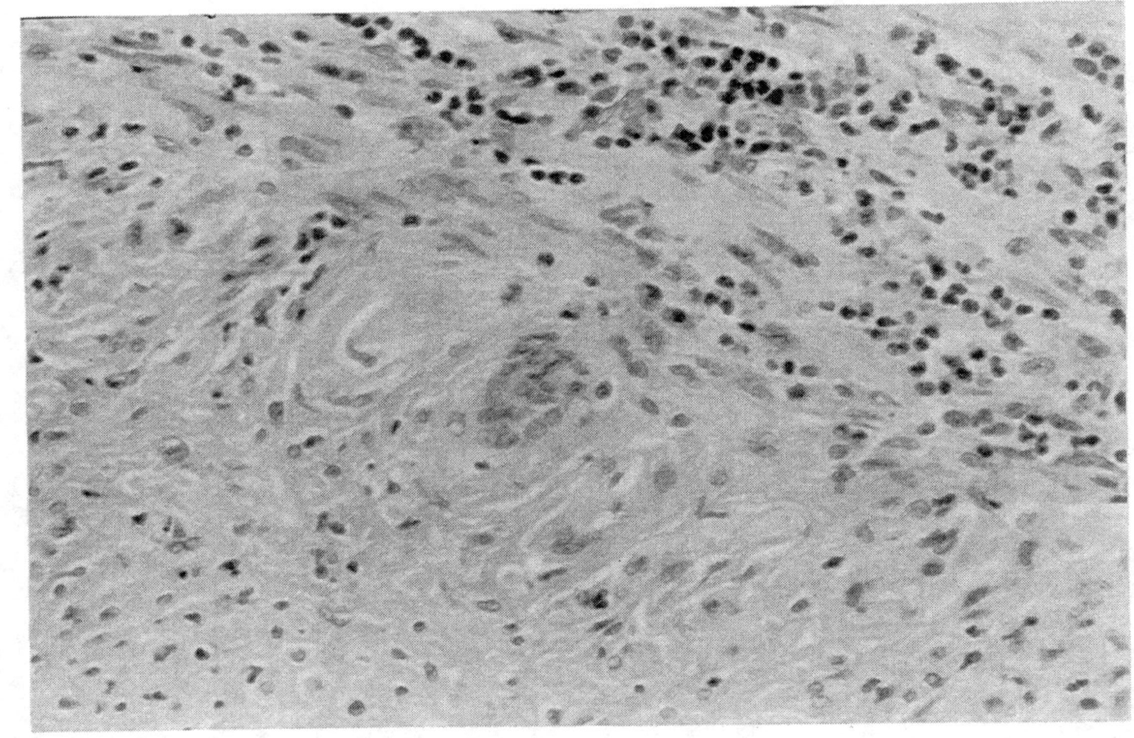

Figure 6B. A higher magnification of the same vessel showing the nature of the inflammatory infiltrate including a multinucleated giant cell, histiocytes and lymphocytes. (H&E x200)

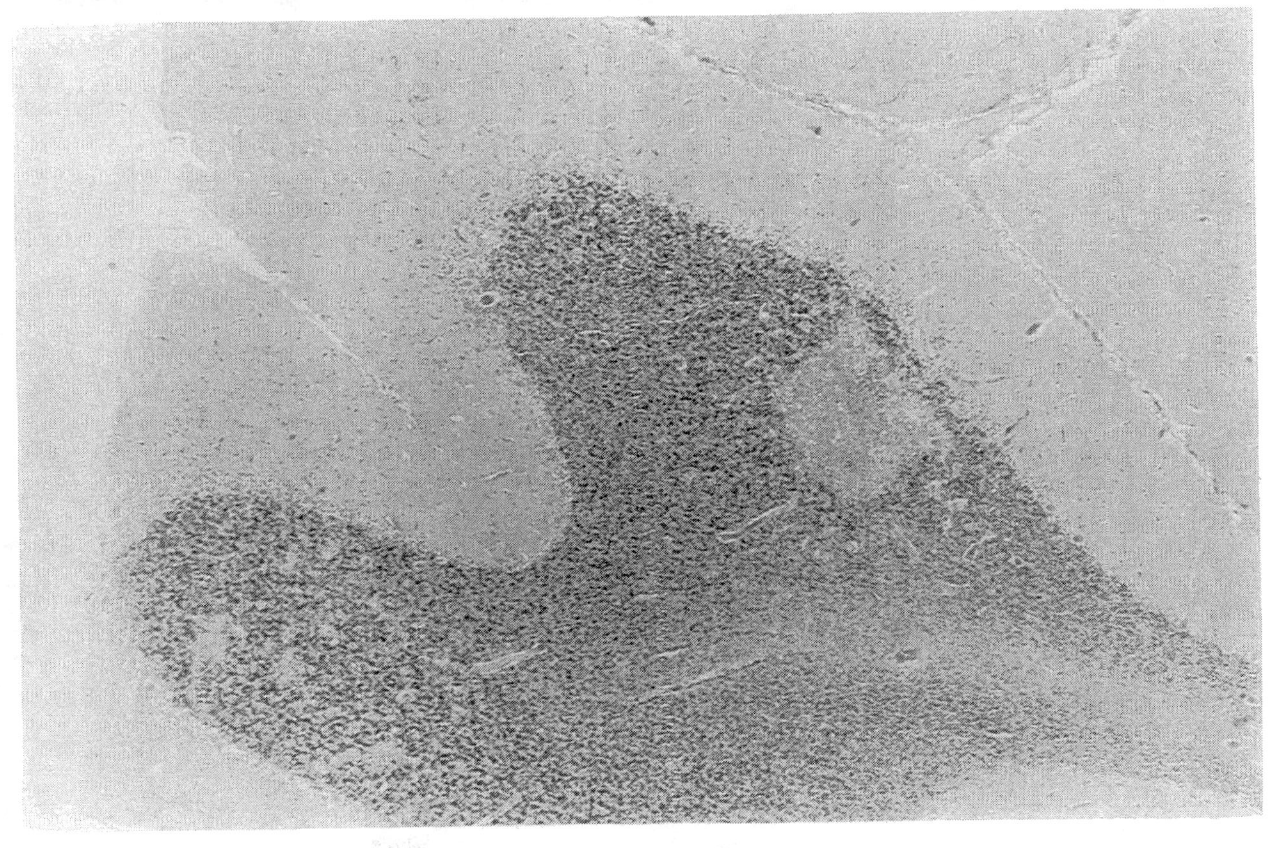

Figure 7A. A case of thrombotic microangiopathy showing microinfarctions in the internal granular layer of the cerebellum. (H&E x40)

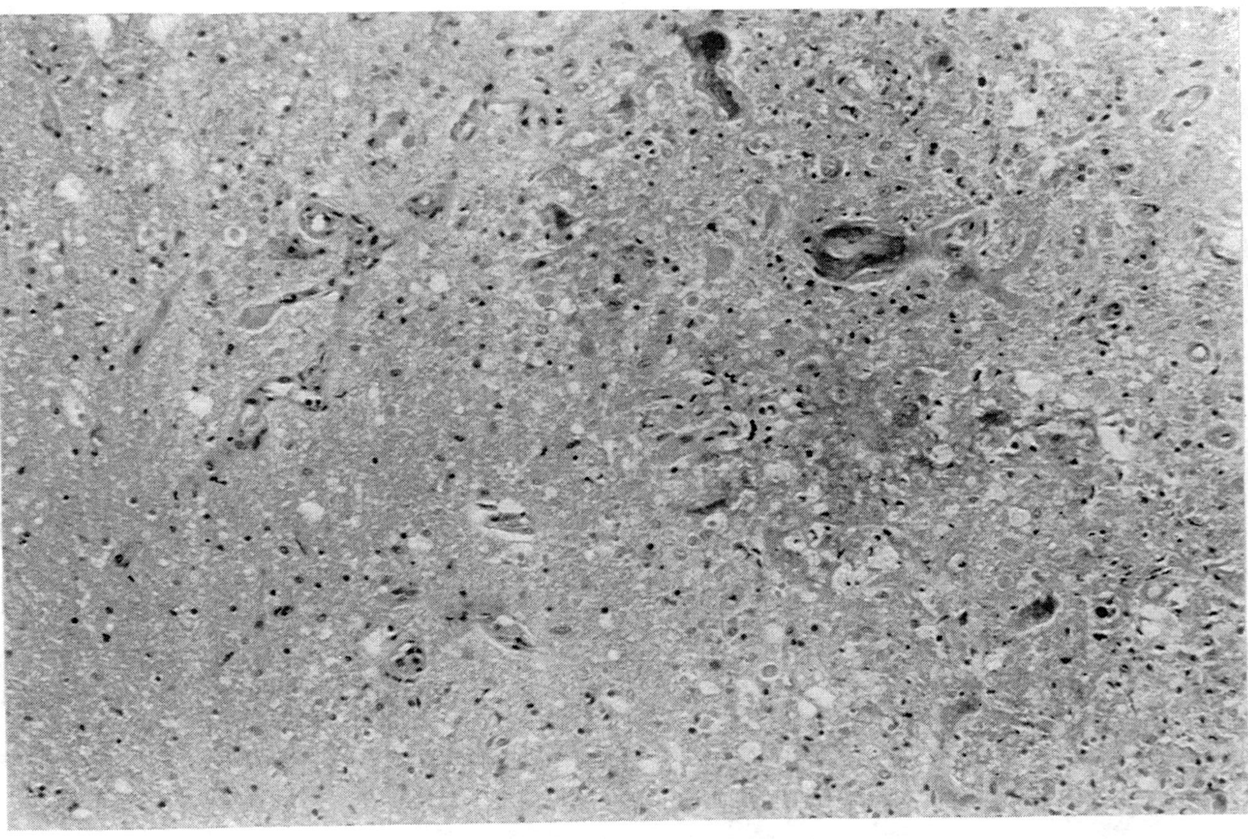

Figure 7B. A section from the dentate nucleus of the same patient showing microinfarctions, thrombosed capillaries and small arterioles, and proliferation of capillaries. (H&E x200).

REFERENCES

1.   Brierley, J.B. and D.I. Graham, Hypoxia and vascular disorders of the central nervous system, in *Greenfield's Neuropathology*, J.H. Adams, J.A.N. Corsellis, and L.W. Duchen, Editor. 1984, John Wiley & Sons: New York NY. p. 125-207.

2.   Brown, A.W. and J.B. Brierley, Evidence for early anoxic-ischemic cell damage in the rat brain. *Experientia*, 1966. 22: p. 546-547.

3.   Brierley, J.B., A.W. Brown, and B.S. Meldrum, The nature and the time course of the neuronal alterations resulting from oligaemia and hypoglycemia in the brain of Macaca mulatta. *Brain Research*, 1971. 25: p. 483-499.

4.   Brown, A.W., Structural abnormalities in neurons. *J. Clin. Pathol.*, 1977. 30 (Suppl): p. 155-169.

5.   Brown, A.W. and J.B. Brierley, The nature, distribution, and earliest stages of anoxic-ischemic nerve damage in the rat brain as defined by the optical microscope. *Brit. J. Exper. Pathol.*, 1968. 49: p. 87-106.

6.   Brown, A.W. and J.B. Brierley, The earliest alterations in rat neurons after anoxia-ischemia. *Acta. Neuropathol.*, 1973. 23: p. 9-22.

7.   Levy, D.E., J.B. Brierley, and F. Plum, Ischemic brain damage in the gerbil in the absence of "no-reflow", *J. Neurol. Neurosurg. Psychiat.*, 1975. 38: p. 1197-1205.

8.   Lindenberg, R., Compression of brain arteries as a pathogenic factor for tissue necrosis and their area of predilection. *J. Neuropath. Exper. Neurol.*, 1955. 14: p. 223-243.

9.   Lindenberg, R., Patterns of CNS vulnerability in acute hypoxemia, including anesthetic accidents, in *Selective vulnerability of the brain in hypoxemia*, J.P. Schade and W.H. McMenemey, Editor. 1963, Blackwell Scientific: Oxford. p. 184-209.

10.   Meyer, A., Neuropathological aspects of anoxia. *Proceed. Roy. Soc. Med.*, 1956. 49: p. 619-622.

11.   Little, J.R., T.M. Sundt, and F.W.L. Kerr, Neuronal alterations in developing cortical infarction. An experimental study in monkeys. *J. Neurosurg.*, 1974. 39: p. 186-198.

12.   Pulsinelli, W.A., J.B. Brierley, and F. Plum, Temporal profile of neuronal damage in a model of transient forebrain ischemia. *Ann. Neurol.*, 1982. 11: p. 491-498.

13.   Rorke, L.B., Differential vulnerability of developing brain to hypoxia, in Pathology of perinatal brain injury. 1982, Raven Press: New York. p. 4-12.

14.   Meyer, A., Anoxias, intoxications and metabolic disorders, in *Greenfield's Neuropathology*, W. Blackwood, et al., Editor. 1963, Williams and Wilkins: Baltimore, Maryland. p. 235-287.

15.   Connett, M.C. and J.M. Lausche, Fibromuscular hyperplasia of the internal carotid artery. Report of a case. *Ann. Surg.*, 1965. 162: p. 59-62.

16.   Luscher, T.F., et al., Arterial fibromuscular dysplasia. *Mayo Clin. Proc.*, 1987. 62: p. 931-952.

17.   Jorens, P.G., et al., Takayasu's disease and atherosclerosis. *J. Cardiovasc. Surg.*, 1991. 32: p. 373-375.

18.   Harrison, C.V., Giant cell or temporal arteritis: a review. *J. Clin. Pathol.*, 1948. 1: p. 197-211.

19.   Heptinstall, R.H., K.H. Porter, and H. Barkley, Giant cell (temporal arteritis). *J. Pathol. Biochem.*, 1954. 67: p. 507-519.

20.   Nordborg, E., B.A. Bengtsson, and C. Nordborg, Temporal artery morphology and morphometry in giant cell arteritis. *APMIS*, 1991. 99: p. 1013-1023.

21.   Walton, E.W., Giant cell granuloma of the respiratory tract (Wegener's granulomatosis). *Br. Med. J.*, 1958. 2: p. 265-270.

22.   Stern, G., Wegener's granulomatosis, in *Handbook of Clinical Neurology. Neurological manifestations of systemic diseases.*, P.J. Vinken and G.W. Bruyn, Editor. 1980, North-Holland: Amsterdam. p. 343-345.

23.   Richardson, E.P., Systemic lupus erythematosus, in *Handbook of Clinical Neurology. Neurological manifestations of systemic diseases*, P.J. Vinken and G.W. Bruyn, Editor. 1980, North-Holland: Amsterdam. p. 283-293.

24.   Adams, R.D., J. Cammermeyer, and P.J. Fitzgerald, Neuropathological aspects of thrombocytic acro-angiothrombosis; clinico-anatomical study of generalized platelet thrombosis. *J. Neurol. Neurosurg. Psychiatr.*, 1948. 11: p. 27-43.

25.   Dawson, T.M., et al., Thrombotic microangiopathy isolated to the central nervous system. *Ann. Neurol.*, 1991. 30: p. 843-846.

26.   Younger, D.S., et al., Granulomatous angiitis of the brain. An inflammatory reaction of diverse etiology. *Arch. Neurol.*, 1988. 45: p. 514-518.

27.   Lie, J.T., Angiitis of the central nervous system. *Curr. Opin. Rheumatol.*, 1991. 3: p. 36-45.

28.   Reyes, M.G., et al., Virus-like particles in granulomatous angiitis of the central nervous system. *Neurology*, 1976. 26: p. 797-799.

29.   Mandybur, T.I., Cerebral amyloid angiopathy: the vascular pathology and complications. *J. Neuropath. Exp. Neurol.*, 1986. 45: p. 79-90.

30.   Vinters, H.V., Cerebral amyloid angiopathy. A critical review. *Stroke*, 1987. 18: p. 311-324.

31.   Frangione, B., Systemic and cerebral amyloidosis. *Ann. Int. Med.*, 1989. 21: p. 69-72.

32.   Haan, J. and R.A. Roos, Amyloid in central nervous system disease. *Clin. Neurol. Neurosurg.*, 1990. 92: p. 305-310.

33.   Jensson, O., et al., The saga of cystatin C gene mutation causing amyloid angiopathy and brain hemorrhage--clinical genetics in Iceland. *Clin. Genet.*, 1989. 36: p. 368-377.

Subject Index